Onychomycosis

the current approach to diagnosis and therapy

Robert Baran, MD
Nail Disease Center,
Cannes, France

Roderick Hay, MD
Professor of Cutaneous Medicine
St John's Institute of Dermatology
St Thomas' Hospital
London, U.K.

Eckart Haneke, MD
Professor and Director
Department of Dermatology
Ferdinand Sauerbruch Hospital
Wuppertal, Germany

Antonella Tosti, MD
Associate Professor of Dermatology
Department of Dermatology
University of Bologna
Bologna, Italy

Bianca Maria Piraccini, MD
Department of Dermatology
University of Bologna
Bologna, Italy

Although every effort has been made to ensure that drug
doses and other information are presented accurately
in this publication, the ultimate responsibility rests with
the prescribing physician. Neither the publishers nor the
authors can be held responsible for errors or for any
consequences arising from the use of information
contained herein.

©R. Baran 1999

First published in the United Kingdom in 1999 by
Martin Dunitz Ltd.
The Livery House
7-9 Pratt Street
London NW1 0AE

Reprinted with corrections 2001

Graphic design by Atelier Höhne, Gräfelfing, Germany
Printed and bound in Spain

A CIP catalogue record for this book is available from the
British Library

ISBN 1-85317-767-9

Robert Baran
Roderick Hay
Eckart Haneke
Antonella Tosti
with the collaboration of Bianca Maria Piraccini

Onychomycosis
the current approach to diagnosis and therapy

Martin Dunitz Ltd.
Publishers

Contents

Preface

This book is written by clinicians for clinicians. In it the authors, who have an abiding interest in all fields of nail pathology, have focused on one of the commonest of nail disorders, onychomycosis. The stepwise approach provides a basis for identifying the most appropriate cost-benefit considerations in the management of fungal nail infection. Consideration of the subject follows a logical path from clinical expression through laboratory diagnosis to therapy. The new classification of the clinical appearances reflects the underlying nail pathology and provides a rational explanation for the pathogenesis and the response to treatment. Compared with the situation ten years ago, there is now a wide choice of treatment options for patients with onychomycosis from topical antifungal agents to nail surgery. The development of new treatment regimens, however, has had the greatest impact on the success of therapy. This in turn has opened the possibility of successful treatment to the majority of patients with fungal nail infections, particularly those caused by dermatophytes. The result has been a major increase in the numbers of patients with onychomycosis presenting for treatment. We hope that this book will provide an up to date review of this common clinical problem which will be of interest to a wide group of health professionals including dermatologists, general practitioners, practice nurses and chiropodists/podiatrists.

The authors

Epidemiology

Onychomycoses are the most common of nail diseases. They occur worldwide, but with variable frequency depending on different climatic, professional and socio-economic conditions. One hundred years ago, they were considered to be very rare, affecting mainly those caring for children with tinea capitis, but their prevalence has increased dramatically during the last few decades (Table 1.1) [1].

Table 1.1
Proportion of onychomycoses to dermatomycoses (literature survey; from [1])

City and year		%
Paris	1910	0.2
Munich	1913–1922	0.13
Berlin	1919–1934	2
Munich	1938	2.6
Hamburg	1938	2.8
Hamburg	1949	10
Munich	1951	8.4
Berlin	1951–1956	17.1
Munich	1958	11.1
Brussels	1980	30

Approximately 1.5% to 15% of persons presenting to a dermatologist have onychomycosis [2, Klein, pers oral comm]. Other estimates suggest between 2% [3] and 23% [4]. There are considerable differences in the prevalence: a survey of 20,000 persons from North Malawi found no onychomycosis though there was a 1.5 to 2.5% prevalence of dermatophytosis in this population [5]; this is probably due to the fact that many of the people do not wear shoes. The frequency of onychomycosis in rural Zaire was 0.89%, but 4% of men and 2.8% of women in towns had fungal nail infections [6]. Large scale studies from Europe, the Middle East and North America have revealed very high rates of fungal nail infections (Table 1.2). A prevalence of 27% was found in coal miners; heat, humidity and common shower facilities were held responsible for this high proportion [7]. In another study carried out 10 years later, 327 out of 1000 people from the Ruhr area in Germany were found to have a dermatophyte infection of their nails [8].

The frequency of onychomycosis increases with age. Although these infections are very rare in young children – two studies found 0.2%, other studies have failed to find a single case and the latest revealed an overall prevalence of 0.44% [16-20, 51] – they are common in young adults and very common in the elderly [19]. Among adolescents, young males are more frequently affected than females; this is probably due to a higher frequency of nail damage due to sports and leisure activities amongst male adolescents. A recent survey among National Basketball Association and Women's National Basketball Association (WNBA) teams found 89% of the players suffered from onychomycosis during their career [19a]. A previous survey in Ohio, USA, showed that approximately 14% of the general population had fungal nail infection and 48% of people >70 years [15].

Eighteen to 40% of all nail diseases are due to fungal infections [21, 22] and approximately 30% of all dermatomycoses are nail infections [2].

By far the most common pathogens are dermatophytes. Virtually unknown in Western Europe at the beginning of the 20th century *Trichophyton rubrum* was probably introduced from West Africa or Asia and has become the most frequent pathogen in Western Europe, North America, and Asia causing 50% to 75% of all cases of onychomycosis [23, 24]. *T. rubrum* and *T. mentagrophytes* together make up at least 80% of onychomycosis in Central Europe [25]. Yeasts can be cultured from 5% to 17% of cases with >70% of these being *Candida albicans* [26]. Non-dermatophyte moulds are considered pathogenic in less than 5% of cases [25, 27-30] and even this proportion is debatable [31]. *Scytalidium dimidiatum, S. hyalinum* and *Scopulariopsis brevicaulis* though are generally accepted as nail pathogens as well as some *Aspergillus, Fusarium, Acremonium* spp and *Onychocola canadensis* [32]. However, there are considerable variations according to geographical location [33]: up to 50% of the onychomycosis cases among Thai conscripts were due to *Scytalidium dimidiatum (Hendersonula toruloidea)* [34]. In Saudi Arabia, most cases of onychomycosis were due to *Candida albicans* with 204 of 243 culturally positive cases of onychomycosis and 241 of 257 cases secondary to paronychia [35]. However in one study 60% of nails that had either been

Table 1.2
Prevalence of onychomycoses world-wide

Country	Year publ	Prevalence [%]	Subjects examined	Authors
Germany	1965	27	Coal miners	7
Britain	1966	2		3
East Germany	1966	13		4
USA	1972	>15–20	Estimate	9
Germany – Ruhr area	1974	32.7	1000 persons	8
Zaire (Congo)	1977	0.9 2.8 4.0	rural areas urban areas – female – male	4 6
Great Britain	1992	2.7	omnibus survey	10
Spain	1995	2.6	computer-assisted telephone interview system	11
Greece	1995	2.5 11.7	fingernails toenails	12
Finland	1995	8.4 11.3 4.3 13	all ages adults females males	19
North Malawi	1996	0	20,000 rural area	5
Great Britain	1996	11	100 diabetics	13
Ontario, Canada	1997	6.9		14
Ohio, USA	1997	14	general population	15
Canada & USA	1997	0,44	2500 children and 50 adolescents under 18 years	20

negative on microscopy or had grown yeasts yielded dermatophytes after nail avulsion [36]. This suggests that growth by contaminant fungi may obscure the presence of the true pathogen. Furthermore, a change in the pattern of fungal pathogens has also been noted during the last decade [37].

Toenails are about seven times more frequently affected than fingernails. The reason for this is probably the growth rate which is about three times slower for toenails than fingernails [32].

The enormous increase in the prevalence of onychomycosis has been attributed to various factors. Increased and prolonged exposure to fungal pathogens through communal bathing and showering facilities, health spas, saunas, and gyms, sports activities, wearing of occlusive footwear, ageing of the population,

increasing numbers of diabetics, administration of immunosuppressive and cytotoxic drugs, and the AIDS epidemic are all thought to predispose to fungal nail infections [38, 39]. However, a series of investigations from France showed that although the main fungal pathogen isolated from public sports facilities was *T. mentagrophytes* the fungi isolated from the feet of the users were mostly *T. rubrum* [40]. Another study from Wales also did not support the assumption that frequent use of public changing facilities is necessarily related to the transmission of fungal infection. Instead, the fact that a high proportion of parents was affected suggested that they might act as the source of infection [17]. Investigations of families from Italy, France and the USA suggest that susceptibility to fungal nail infections, particularly those due to *T. rubrum*, might be inherited as an autosomal dominant trait [41].

Epidemiology

Damaged nails are more susceptible to onychomycoses [3, 42]. This is supported by the observation that dermatophytes can be grown from normal toenails and dermatophyte onycholysis of the big toenail may heal after correction of an underlying foot deformity [43, 44]. Tinea unguium was seen in 42% of subjects with arterial circulatory disorders [45]. Nail changes alone were seen in 8%, and nail and interdigital abnormalities in an additional 22% of vascular disease patients (controls 4% and 0%, respectively). However, cultures were positive in only 9% of patients and 1% of controls [46] (Table 1.3). The role of diabetes mellitus is debatable [47]. There may not be an increased incidence of dermatophyte infections of the nail unit in diabetics but *Candida* infections may be more prevalent [48]. However, for some authorities [49], after controlling for age and sex, the risk ratio in 55 diabetic subjects for onychomycosis of the toes (present in 26.2% of the samples) was 2.77 times greater than that of normal individuals. The majority of organisms implicated in causing onychomycosis were dermatophytes (88%), with *Candida* species in 3% and non-dermatophyte moulds accounting for 9% [49].

Psoriasis and hereditary palmoplantar keratoses also appear to favour fungal nail infections [8, 50-52].

Table 1.3
Frequency of onychomycoses and importance of predisposing diseases

Condition	Number examined	Onycho-mycosis [%]		Reference
Abnormal toenails	72	43		3
Subungual hyperkeratoses	183	34		3
Podiatric	168	37		3
Impaired arterial circulation	112	42		45
Venous insufficiency	100	10 (30)	culture-proven (altered nails)	46
Diabetes mellitus	100	12 to 26		13 & 49
Psoriasis	100	14 16 16	dermatophytes *Candida* spp moulds	8
Psoriasis	120	35 24 15	all fungi dermatophytes *Candida albicans*	50
Psoriasis	78	27 23 30	all nails in psoriatics normal appearing nails altered nails	51
Psoriasis	561 (298 (263	13 0.7 27	all nails normal appearing nails) clinically abnormal nails)	14
Keratosis palmoplantaris				52
Old age (> 70 yrs)		48		15

References

1. Haneke E. Epidemiology and pathology of onychomycoses. In Nolting S, Korting HC, eds. Onychomycoses. Berlin, Springer, 1989:1–8

2. Achten G, Wanet-Rouard J. Onychomycosis (Mycology No. 5). Brussels; Cilag; 1981

3. Walshe MM, English MP. Fungi in nails. Br J Dermatol 1966; 78:198–207

4. Seebacher C. Untersuchungen über die Pilzflora kranker und gesunder Zehennägel. Mykosen 1966; 11:893–902

5. Pönninghaus JM, Clayton Y, Warndorff D. The spectrum of dermatophytes in northern Malawi (Africa). Mycoses 1996; 39:293–297

6. Vanbreuseghem R. Prévalence des onychomycoses au Zaïre particulièrement chez les coupeurs de canne à sucre. Ann Soc Belg Méd Trop 1977; 57:7–15

7. Götz H, Hantschke D. Einblicke in die Epidemiologie der Dermatolmykosen im Kohlenbergbau. Hautarzt 1965, 16:543

8. Götz H, Patiri C, Hantschke D. Das Wachstum von Dermatophyten auf normalem und psoriatischem Nagelkeratin. Mykosen 1974; 17:373–377

9. Zaias N. Onychomycosis. Arch Dermatol 1972; 105:263

10. Roberts DT. Prevalence of dermatophyte onychomycosis in the United Kingdom: results of an omnibus survey. Br J Dermatol 1992; 126: Suppl 39:23–27

11. Sais G, Jucgla A, Peyri J. Prevalence of dermatophyte onychomycosis in Spain: a cross-sectional study. Br J Dermatol 1995; 132:758–61

12. Devliotou-Panagiotidou D, Koussidou-Eremondi T, Badillet G. Dermatophytosis in northern Greece during the decade 1981–1990. Mycoses 1995; 38:151–157

13. Buxton PK, Milne LJR, Prescott RJ, Proudfoots MC; Stuart FM. The prevalence of dermatophyte infection in well-controlled diabetics and the response to Trichophyton antigens. Br J Dermatol 1996; 134:900–903

14. Gupta AK, Lynde CW, Jain HC, Sibbald RG, Elewski BE, Daniel CR III, Watteel GN, Summerbell RC. A higher prevalence of onychomycosis in psoriatics compared with non-psoriatics: a multicentre study. Br J Dermatol 1997; 136:786–789

15. Elewski B & Charif MA. Prevalence of onychomycosis in patients attending a dermatology clinic in northeastern Ohio for other conditions. Arch Dermatol 1997; 133: 1172–1173

16. Findlay GH, Vismar HF, Sophianos T. Spectrum of paediatric dermatology. Br J Dermatol 1974; 91:379–387

17. Philpot CM, Shuttleworth D. Dermatophyte onychomycosis in children. Clin Exp Dermatol 1989; 14:203–205

18. Khosravi AR, Aghamirian MR, Mahmoudi M. Dermatophytoses in Iran. Mycoses 1994; 37:43–48

19. Heikkilä H, Stubb S. The prevalence of onychomycosis in Finland. Br J Dermatol 1995; 133:699–703

19a. McNerney J. Onychomycosis in special populations (SS02-05). JEADV 2000; 14 (suppl 14), 83.

20. Gupta AK, Sibbald RG, Lynde CD, Hull PR, Shear NH, de Doncker P, Daniel CR III. Onychomycosis in children: prevalence and treatment strategies. J Am Acad Dermatol 1997; 36:395–402

21. Langer H. Epidemiologische und klinische Untersuchungen bei Onychomykosen. Arch Klin Exp Dermatol 1957; 204:624

22. Achten G, Wanet-Rouard J. Onychomycosis in the laboratory. Mykosen 1978; 23, Suppl 1:125

23. Dardé ML. Epidémiologie des dermatophyties. Ann Dermatol Vénéréol 1992; 119:99–100

24. Manzano-Gayosso P, Méndez-Tovar LJ, Hernández-Hernández F, López-Martínez R. Dermatophytoses in Mexico City. Mycoses 1994; 37:49–52

25. Clayton YM. Clinical and mycological diagnostic aspects of onychomycoses and dermatomycoses. Clin Exp Dermatol 1992; 17: suppl 1:37–40

26. Cohen J, Scher RK, Pappert A. The nail and fungus infections. In Elewski B, ed. Cutaneous Fungal Infections. New York, Igaku Shoin, 1992:106–123

27. Summerbell RC, Kane J, Krajden S. Onychomycosis, tinea pedis, and tinea manuum caused by non-dermatophytic filamentous fungi. Mycoses 1989; 32:609–619

28. Willemsen MD. Changing pattern in superficial infections: focus on onychomycosis. J Eur Acad Dermatol Venereol 1995; 2:S6–S11

29. Williams HC. The epidemiology of onychomycosis in Britain. Br J Dermatol 1993; 129:101–109

30. Greer DL. Etiology of onychomycosis: review of the literature. Issues in the modern management of onychomycosis. Monte Carlo 1993

31. Ellis DH, Watson AB, Marley JE, Williams TG. Non-dermatophytes in onychomycosis of the toenails. Br J Dermatol 1997; 136:490–493

32. Haneke E. Fungal infections of the nail. Sem Dermatol 1991; 10: 41–53

33. Elewski BE, Hay RJ. Update on the management of onychomycosis: Highlights of the Third Annual International Summit of Cutaneous Antifungal Therapy. Clin Inf Dis 1996; 23:305–313

34. Kotrajaras R, Chongsathein S, Rojanavanich V, Buddhavudhikarai P, Viriyayadhakorn S. Hendersonula toruloidea infection in Thailand. Int J Dermatol 1988; 27:391–395

35. Al-Sogair SM, Moawad MK, Al-Humaidan YM. Fungal infection as a cause of skin disease in the Eastern Province of Saudi Arabia: prevailing fungi and pattern of infection. Mycoses 1991; 34:333–337

36. Szili M, Sándor L. Comparative mycological studies from nails removed because of onychomycosis (Hungarian). Börgyógy Venerol Szle 1984; 60:175–177

37. Ginter G, Rieger E, Heigl K, Propst E. Steigende Häufigkeit der Onychomykose – Ändert sich das Erregerspektrum? Mycoses 1996; 39: Suppl 1:118–122

38. Barranco V. New approaches to the diagnosis and management of onychomycosis. Int J Dermatol 1994; 33:292–299

39. Conant MA. The AIDS epidemic. J Am Acad Dermatol 1994; 31: Suppl:S47–S50

40. Feuilhade M. Pied et mycoses. Aspects épidémiologiques. Pied 1990; 6:5–6

41. Zaias N, Tosti A, Rebell G, Morelli R, Bardazzi F, Bieley H, Zaiac M, Glick B, Paley B; Allevato M, Baran R. Autosomal dominant pattern of distal subungual onychomycosis caused by Trichophyton rubrum. J Am Acad Dermatol 1996; 34:302–304

42. Male O, Tappeiner J. Nagelveränderungen durch Schimmelpilze. Dermatol Wschr 1965; 151–212

43. Baran R, Badillet G. Un dermatophyte unguéal est-il nécessairement pathogène? Ann Dermatol Vénérérol 1983; 110:629–631

44. Baran R, Badillet G. Primary onycholysis of the big toenail: a review of 112 cases. Br J Dermatol 1982; 106:529–534

45. Dahlke H. Zur Pathogenese der Tinea pedis, insbesondere bei peripheren Durchblutungsstörungen. Mykosen 1971; 14:409–413

46. Wienert V, Stemmer R. Onychomykosen bei phlebologischen Patienten. Phlebol Proktol 1982; 11:281–283

47. Buxton PK; Milne LJR, Prescott RJ et al.. The prevalence of dermatophyte infection in well-controlled diabetics and the response to Trichophyton antigen. Br J Dermatol. 1996; 134: 900–903

48. Rich P. Special patient populations: onychomycosis in the diabetic patient. J Am Acad Dermatol. 1996; 35:S10–S12

49. Gupta AK, Konnikof N, Mac Donald P et al. Prevalence and epidermiology of toenail onychomycosis in diabetic subjects: a multicentre survey. Br J Dermatol 1998; 139: 665–671

50. Feuerman E, Alteras I, Aryelly J. The incidence of pathogenic fungi in psoriatic nails. Castellania 1976; 4:195–196

51. Staberg B, Gammeltoft MD, Onsberg P. Onychomycosis in patients with psoriasis. Acta Dermatol Venereol 1983; 63: 436–438

52. Nielsen PG, Faergemann J. Dermatophytes and keratin in patients with hereditary palmoplantar keratoderma. Acta Dermatol Venereol 1993; 73:416–418

The nail unit lies immediately above the periostium of the distal phalanx and consists of a keratinized product, the nail plate, and four specialized epithelia : the proximal nail fold (or eponychium), the nail matrix, the nail bed and the hyponychium (Fig 2.1) [1, 2].

Nail plate

The nail plate is a fully keratinized multilayered sheet of cornified cells. From the 15th week of embryonic life, nail plate production occurs continuously and thereafter almost uniformly throughout life [1]. The nail plate is almost rectangular in shape and translucent. It appears pink because of the blood vessels of the underlying nail bed. The nail plate adheres tightly to the nail bed, since the horny layer of the nail bed partially contributes to the formation of the ventral nail plate [3]. The nail plate has a somewhat loose attachment, along its lateral borders [4].

Fig 2.1
Sagittal section
through fingernail

Transverse section
through fingernail

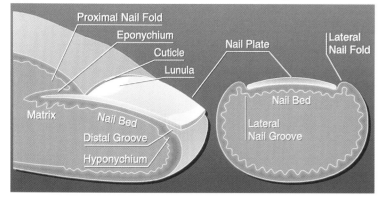

Proximally and laterally, the nail plate is surrounded by the proximal and lateral folds, whereas its distal margin is free. Detachment of the nail plate from the underlying tissues occurs at the hyponychium, which marks the separation of the nail from the digit. The nail plate's free edge appears white due the presence of air in the subungual space.This space frequently contains keratinous debris, especially in the toenails.

The proximal part of the fingernails, especially the thumbs, shows a whitish, opaque, half-moon-shaped area, the lunula, which is the visible portion of the nail matrix. The shape of the lunula determines the shape of the free edge of the nail plate.

More than 90% of fingernails show a thin distal transverse white band, the onychocorneal band, which marks the most distal portion of firm attachment of the nail plate to the nail bed [5]. This area represents an important anatomical barrier against environmental and microbial hazards.

In transverse sections, the nail plate consists of three portions : dorsal nail plate, intermediate nail plate and ventral nail plate [6]. The dorsal and intermediate portions of the nail plate are produced by the nail matrix and consist of hard keratins. The intermediate nail plate, which is produced by the distal matrix, represents ⅔ of the whole nail thickness. The ventral portion of the nail plate is produced by the nail bed and is formed by soft keratins. The thickness of this portion of the nail plate considerably increases in nail bed disorders.

Nail matrix

The nail matrix consists of a proliferative epithelium that keratinizes in the absence of a granular layer. Maturation and differentiation of nail matrix keratinocytes lead to the formation of the superficial and intermediate layers of the nail plate. The site of nail matrix keratinization can be recognized in histological sections as an eosinophilic band (keratogenous zone). In this area, nail matrix keratinocytes show nuclear fragmentation and condensation of cytoplasm.

In longitudinal sections the matrix consists of a proximal (dorsal) and a distal (ventral) region. Proximal nail matrix keratinocytes give rise to the upper portion of the nail plate whereas distal nail matrix keratinocytes produce its intermediate portion.

The nail matrix epithelium contains melanocytes. Although nail matrix melanocytes are usually quiescent, they may start to produce melanin in a large number of physiological and pathological conditions. This is more common in Black and Asian populations than in Caucasians. The nail growth rates range from 1.8 to 4.8 mm/month in fingernails and 1.3 to 1.8 mm/month in toenails. This gradually declines with age [7]. Complete replacement of a fingernail requires 4 to 6 months and that of a toenail 12 to 18 months. Linear nail growth may also increase in some physiological and pathological circumstances and may be influenced by drugs. The triazole derivatives itraconazole [8] and fluconazole [9] have been reported to enhance nail growth. Terbinafine may also induce an increase of linear nail growth [10].

Nail bed

The nail bed epithelium consists of several cell layers and extends from the lunula to the hyponychium. Nail bed keratinization occurs in the absence of a granular layer and gives rise to the ventral nail plate. This corresponds to about 1/5 of the terminal nail thickness and it can be recognized in histological sections because of its mild eosinophilia.

The nail bed dermoepidermal architecture shows a distinctive arrangement, with longitudinal grooves and ridges extending from the lunula to the hyponychium. The nail bed capillaries run longitudinally along these nail bed grooves.

The nail bed epithelium is so adherent to the nail plate that it remains attached to the undersurface of the nail when this is avulsed.

Hyponychium

The hyponychium is normally covered by the nail plate's free margin, but becomes visible in nail biters or when the nail plate is cut very short.

Its epithelium is similar to that of plantar or volar skin and it keratinizes through the formation of a granular layer. Cornified hyponychial cells accumulate in the subungual space, especially in toenails.

Proximal nail fold

The proximal nail plate is surrounded and partially covered by the proximal nail fold, which overlies about a quarter of the nail plate. Adhesion between proximal nail fold and nail plate is tight due to the presence of the cuticle, which is firmly attached to the superficial nail plate. The cuticle, which is continuously formed by keratinization of the proximal nail plate, consists of a thin layer of orthokeratotic cells.

The proximal nail fold consists of a dorsal portion that is anatomically similar to the skin of the dorsum of the digit and a ventral portion that continues proximally with the proximal matrix.

References

1. Zaias N. The nail in health and disease, 2nd ed. Appleton & Lange, Norwalk, 1990.
2. Baran R, Dawber RPR. Disease of the nails and their management. Blackwell, Oxford, 1994.
3. Johnson M, Cosmaish JS, Shuster S. Nail is produced by the normal nail bed : a controversy resolved. Br J Dermatol. 1991; 125:27–29.

4. Baran R, De Doncker P. Lateral edge involvement indicates poor prognosis for treating onychomycosis with the new systemic antifungals. Acta Derm Venereol. 1996; 73: 82–83.
5. Sonnex TS, Griffiths WAD, Nicol WJ. The nature and significance of the transverse white band of human nails. Seminars Dermatol. 1981; 10: 12–16.
6. Forslind B. Biophysical studies of the normal nail. Acta Derm Venereol. 1970; 50: 161–168.
7. Bean WB. Nail growth. Twenty-five year's observation. Arch Intern Med. 1968; 122: 359–361.

8. De Doncker P, Pierard G. Acquired nail beading in patients receiving itraconazole. An indicator of faster nail growth ? A study using optical profilometry. Clin Exp Derm. 1994; 19: 404–406.
9. Shelley WB, Shelley ED. Portrait of a practice. Cutis 1992; 49: 386.
10. Faergemann J, Anderson C, Hersle K et al. Double-blind, parallel-group comparison of terbinafine and griseofulvin in the treatment of toenail onychomycosis. J Am Acad Dermatol. 1995; 32: 750–753.

3

Clinical patterns correlated with main routes of entry

A fungus gains entry to the nail by four main routes, each resulting in different clinical patterns of infection [1–2]. These are :

● **Via the distal subungual area and the lateral nail groove** (Fig 3.1) leading to distal lateral subungual onychomycosis (DLSO) (Fig 3.2). The fungus invades the horny layer of the hyponychium and/or the nail bed, then the undersurface of the nail plate which becomes opaque. This causes thickening of the horny layer raising the free edge of the nail plate with disruption of the normal nail plate-nail bed attachment. The disease spreads proximally against the stream of nail growth. Sometimes a yellow brown discoloration is observed. *T. rubrum* is the most common fungal invader, *T. mentagrophytes var. interdigitale* is much less common and *Epidermophyton floccosum* is rare. In contrast to this form, DLSO may also appear as primary onycholysis with a minimum of hyperkeratosis especially in fingernails (Fig 3.3). Primary onycholysis may be associated with the presence of *Candida* (Fig 3.4). Overriding of the toes and repeated microtrauma of the nail against the shoes may create an area of onycholysis favourable to the invasion of microorganisms. In such cases, mixed infection due to *T. rubrum* and *Pseudomonas* is not exceptional (Fig 3.5).The clinical significance of nail invasion or colonization by fungi which are not normally pathogenic needs to be carefully considered in the light of laboratory findings.

The nail bed infection in DLSO caused by *T. rubrum* is the result of the fungus spreading from the plantar (Fig 3.6) [3] and palmar surface of the feet and hands, a pattern seen in the one-hand/two-foot tinea syndrome (Fig 3.7) [4].

T. mentagrophytes var. interdigitale produces a chronic syndrome with episodic pruritic vesicles in the skin of the plantar arch and in the toewebs where scaling is also visible. Intermittent vesicles, scaling of the heel and thickening of the skin of the sole are often visible. This syndrome can also be observed in patients with superficial white onychomycosis caused by the same fungus. Organisms such as *Scytalidium dimidiatum* which mimic the pattern of disease caused by dermatophytes produce the clinical pattern of DLSO but this is often associated with onycholysis and, sometimes, paronychia in fingernails (Fig 3.8).

Fig 3.1
Distal lateral subungual onychomycosis

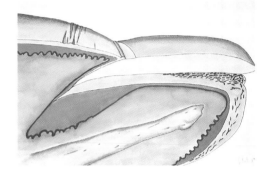

Fig 3.2
DLSO due to *T. rubrum*

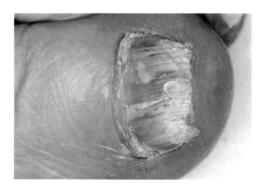

Fig 3.3
DLSO with onycholysis due to *T. rubrum*

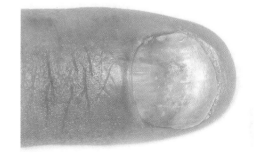

Fig 3.4
Candida onycholysis

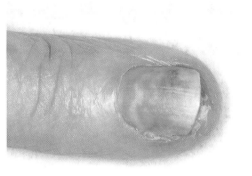

Fig 3.7
One-hand/two-foot syndrome

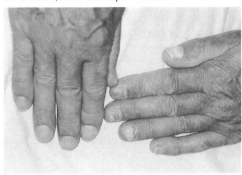

Fig 3.5
Mixed infection due to *T. rubrum*
and *Pseudomonas*

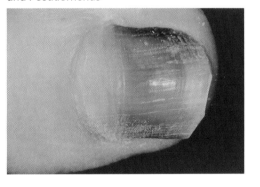

Fig 3.8
DLSO due to *Scytalidium dimidiatum*
with associated paronychia

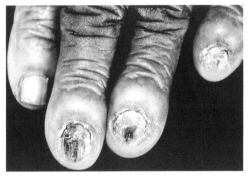

Fig 3.6
Tinea pedis

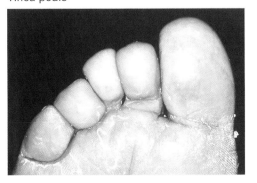

Clinical patterns correlated
with main routes of entry

● **Via the dorsal surface of the nail plate**
(Fig 3.9), producing superficial onychomycosis
(SO) (Fig 3.10). Superficial white onychomycosis (SWO) is normally confined to the
toenails. The causative organisms produce the
clinical picture of small, white patches with
distinct edges on the dorsal nail plate. These
latter coalesce and may gradually cover the
whole nail. The chalky white surface becomes
roughened and the texture softer than normal.
T. mentagrophytes var. interdigitale is responsible for more than 90% of the cases. Lesions
of SWO may range from minimal to extensive
and are part of a syndrome caused by
T. mentagrophytes var. interdigitale that
includes interdigital tinea pedis and vesicular-
arch-type tinea pedis.

Superficial infections caused by non-dermatophyte moulds such as *Aspergillus terreus,
Fusarium oxysporum* or *Acremonium* spp. are
more often seen in patients in tropical and sub-
tropical environments. Children presenting with
SWO may have *Candida albicans* infection .

Superficial black onychomycosis (SBO),
the counterpart of SWO is very rare. Cases
reported have been produced by *T. rubrum* and
Scytalidium dimidiatum (Fig 3.11) [5, 6].

Fig 3.9
Superficial onychomycosis

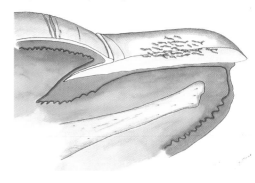

Fig 3.10
Superficial white onychomycosis

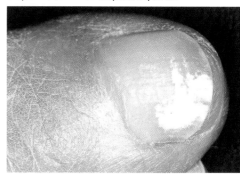

Fig 3.11
Superficial black onychomycosis
due to *Scytalidium dimidiatum*

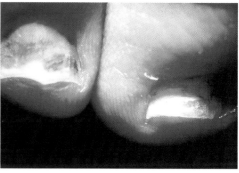

Courtesy CE Meisel (Germany)

● **Via the undersurface of the proximal nail fold** (Fig 3.12), which appears normal, in proximal subungual onychomycosis (PSO) (Fig 3.13).

This variety may affect finger as well as toenails. The stratum corneum of the ventral aspect of the proximal nail fold is the primary site of the fungal invasion. When it reaches the matrix, the fungus mainly invades the lower portion of the nail plate and a white spot appears beneath the cuticle and advances distally.

This type of nail invasion is usually caused by *T. rubrum*. Exceptionally, *T. megninii*, *T. schoenleinii* or *Epidermophyton floccosum* have been reported. Recently proximal subungual onychomycosis without paronychia due to *Candida* has been demonstrated [7].

A rapidly developing form of proximal white subungual onychomycosis (PWSO) has been recorded in patients with acquired immune deficiency syndrome (AIDS) and this is now recognized as a marker for immunodeficient patients [8]. The infection, more frequent when the CD4 (+) cell count is less than 450 cells/mm^3, may spread to all the fingers (even over the paronychium [9]) and toenails. This is caused by preexisting tinea pedis due to *T. rubrum* that predates immunosuppression.

Sometimes, PSO due to *T. rubrum* may extend to the superficial nail plate producing a clinical picture that resembles SWO. This is almost exclusively seen in fingernails, but has also been described in children who have thin toenails [10].

● **PSO secondary to paronychia** (Fig 3.14). Paronychia is observed mainly in adult women and affects particularly the index, middle finger and thumb of the dominant hand. Frequent manual work with carbohydrate-containing foods and moisture, maceration, occlusion, hyperhidrosis and acrocyanosis favour the disease. Diabetes mellitus and other hormonal disturbances and drugs such as corticosteroids, cytotoxics and antibiotics may favour secondary *Candida* infection and exacerbate paronychia. The first step in the development of chronic paronychia is mechanical infection or chemical trauma that produce cuticle damage. At that time the epidermal barrier of the ventral aspect

Fig 3.12
Proximal subungual onychomycosis

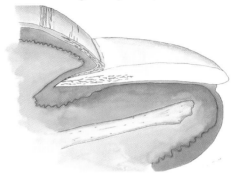

Fig 3.13
Proximal subungual onychomycosis due to *T. rubrum*

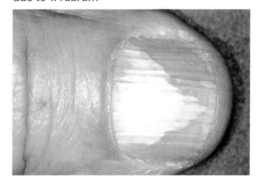

Fig 3.14
Proximal subungual onychomycosis with chronic paronychia

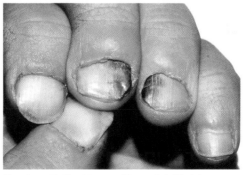

Courtesy S. Goettmann-Bonvallot (Paris)

of the proximal nail fold is destroyed and the area is suddenly exposed to a variety of environmental hazards. Irritants and allergens may then produce an inflammatory reaction of the nail fold and nail matrix, which interferes with the normal nail growth. Usually the nail fold inflammation affects the lateral portion of the matrix leading to nail plate deformity on the same side, appearing as irregular transverse ridging or a dark narrow strip down one or both lateral borders of the nail.

The thickened free end of the erythematous proximal nail fold becomes rounded, retracted and loses the ability to form a cuticle. The disease tends to run a protracted course interrupted by subacute exacerbations due to secondary *Candida* and bacterial infection with formation of a small abscess in the space formed between the proximal nail fold and the nail plate. *Candida* spp. and bacteria are frequently isolated from beneath the proximal nail fold in patients with chronic paronychia [11].

Depending on the major etiological factors involved, chronic paronychia can be classified into the following types [12] :

1. Contact allergy (topical drug ingredients, rubber etc…)

2. Food hypersensitivity (a variety of immediate contact dermatitis due to foods)

3. *Candida* hypersensitivity (a similar reaction to that suggested in some patients with recurrent vaginitis)

4. Irritative reaction (irritative chronic paronychia may subsequently acquire a secondary hypersensitivity and chronic food hypersensitivity paronychia and/or *Candida* hypersensitivity paronychia may develop)

5. *Candida* paronychia.

   True *Candida* paronychia is uncommon in temperate climates except in patients with chronic mucocutaneous candidosis and HIV infection. In this condition proximal nail fold inflammation is usually associated with proximal onycholysis or onychomycosis due to *Candida* which can be isolated both from the proximal nail fold and clippings of the affected nail plate.

   In contrast to *Candida* infection, non-dermatophyte moulds such as *Fusarium* (Fig 3.15) may produce subacute paronychia accompanied by proximal white onychomycosis both in immunocompetent and in immunocompromised individuals [13]. *Scopulariopsis brevicaulis* (Fig 3.16) may be responsible for identical features with a white or yellow discoloration of the nail plate [14]. PSO may also be associated with marked periungual inflammation and black discoloration of the lunula region due to *Aspergillus niger* [15].

6. Bacterial paronychia

   The existence of chronic paronychia solely attributable to bacteria is debatable, although in some patients the only readily identifiable aetiological agents are bacteria, usually Gram negative forms.

Fig 3.15
Proximal subungual onychomycosis due to *Fusarium*

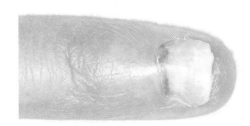

Fig 3.16
Proximal subungual onychomycosis with paronychia due to *Scopulariopsis brevicaulis*

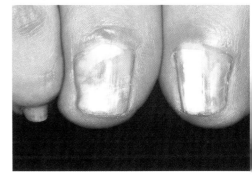

● **Endonyx onychomycosis** (Fig 3.17).
A new form of invasion of the nail plate by fungal elements has been described [16]. The dermatophyte reaches the nail plate via the pulp as in the DLSO type. Instead of infecting the nail bed however, the fungus penetrates the nail keratin where it forms milky white patches without subungual hyperkeratosis or onycholysis. Endonyx infection has been described with *T. soudanense* (Fig 3.18), but may also be due to *T. violaceum* infection. Both dermatophytes

cause endothrix hair shaft invasion in tinea capitis.

● **Total dystrophic onychomycosis** (TDO) (Fig 3.19).
Secondary TDO (Fig 3.20) represents the most advanced form of all the types described above. The nail crumbles and disappears, leaving a thickened, abnormal nail bed retaining keratotic nail debris.

Fig 3.17
Endonyx onychomycosis

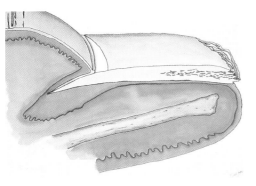

Fig 3.18
Endonyx onychomycosis due to
Trichophyton soudanense

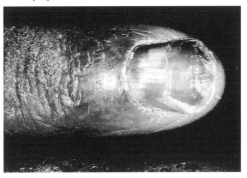

Fig 3.19
Development of total dystrophic onychomycosis

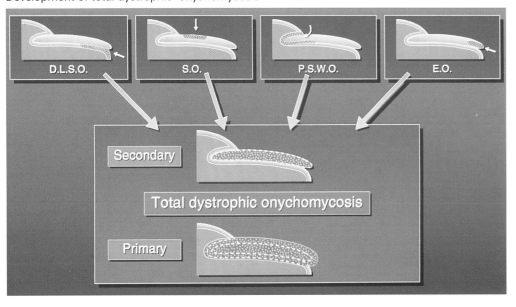

In the new form of total nail dystrophy observed in patients with AIDS, infection appears to have spread from under the proximal nail fold (PSO) but this has not been established in all cases. The dorsum of the nail plate may also be involved. The term acute TDO might be appropriate for this type of infection.

Contrary to secondary TDO, primary TDO is observed only in patients suffering from chronic mucocutaneous candidosis (CMC) (Fig 3.21) or in other immunodeficiency states (see Table 3.1) [17]. *Candida* invasion rapidly involves all the tissues of the nail apparatus. The thickening of the soft tissues results in a swollen distal phalanx more bulbous than clubbed. The nail plate is thickened, opaque and yellow-brown in colour. Hyperkeratotic areas secondary to *Candida* invasion may develop in skin adjacent to the nail. Oral candidosis is generally present in these patients. This syndrome, which usually occurs in childhood or infancy, recurs despite treatment. Dual infection with dermatophytes may occur in patients with CMC.

Fig 3.20
Secondary total dystrophic onychomycosis

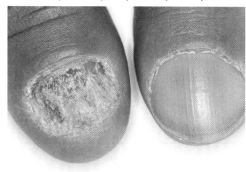

Fig 3.21
Primary total dystrophic onychomycosis

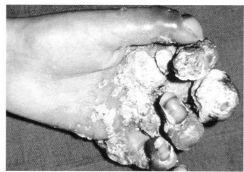

Courtesy D. Leroy (Caen)

Table 3.1
Subtypes of chronic mucocutaneous candidosis (CMC) @ [17] (with permission)

Type	Pattern of inheritance	Special clinical/immunological features
CMC		
Without endocrinopathy (212050)*	Recessive	Childhood onset
With endocrinopathy #(240300)	Recessive	Childhood onset. Patients have the polyendocrinopathy syndrome
Without endocrinopathy (114580)	Dominant	Childhood onset
With endocrinopathy	Dominant	Childhood onset Associated with hypothyroidism
Sporadic CMC	None known	Childhood onset
CMC with keratitis	None known	Childhood onset. Associated with keratitis
Late-onset CMC §	None known	Onset in adult life Associated with thymoma

* McKusick numbers.
@ While originally severe CMC (e.g. *Candida granuloma*) was described in association with specific subtypes it is now apparent that extensive infection, including hyperkeratotic candidiasis and dermatophytosis, is not specific to any one variety.

The main endocrine diseases seen with this variety are hypo-parathyroidism and hypo-adrenalism.
§ Other late-onset types have been recorded e.g. with systemic lupus erythematosus, but as they are usually associated with systemic corticosteroid therapy, they have been excluded as secondary candidosis.

References

1. Zaias N. Onychomycosis. Arch Dermatol. 1972; 105: 263-274
2. Baran R, Hay RJ, Tosti A, Haneke E. A new classification of onychomycosis. Br J Dermatol. 1998; 119: 567-571.
3. Evans EGV. Causative pathogens in onychomycosis and the possibility of treatment resistance: A review. J Am Acad Dermatol. 1998; 38: S 32-36.
4. Daniel CR III, Gupta AK, Daniel MP, Daniel CM. Two feet-one hand syndrome : a retrospective multicenter survey. Int J Dermatol. 1997; 36: 658-660.
5. Badillet G. Mélanonychies superficielles. Bull Soc Fr Mycol Med. 1988; 17: 335-340.
6. Meisel CE, Quadripur SA. Onychomycosis due to *Hendersonula toruloidea*. Hautnah myk 1992; 6: 232-234.

7. Baran R. Proximal subungual Candida onychomycosis. An unusual manifestation of chronic mucocutaneous candidosis. Br J Dermatol. 1997; 137: 286-288.
8. Daniel III CR, Norton LA, Scher RK. The spectrum of nail disease in patients with immunodeficiency virus infection. J Am Acad Dermatol. 1992; 27: 93-97.
9. Kaplan MH, Sadick N, McNutt S et al. Dermatologic findings and manifestations of AIDS. J Am Acad Dermatol. 1987; 16: 485-506.
10. Ploysangan T, Lucky AW. Childhood white superficial onychomycosis caused by Trichophyton rubrum. J Am Acad Dermatol. 1997; 36: 29-32.
11. Daniel CR, Daniel MP, Daniel CM, Sullivan S, Ellis G. Chronic paronychia and onycholysis. A thirteen-year experience. Cutis 1996; 58: 397-401.
12. Tosti A, Piraccini BM. Paronychia. In : Amin S, Maibach HI (eds). Contact urticaria syndrome. CRC Press Boca Raton USA, 1997, Chap 26, p 267-278.

13. Baran R, Tosti A, Piraccini BM. Uncommon clinical patterns of Fusarium nail infection : report of three cases. Br J Dermatol. 1997; 136: 424-427.
14. Tosti A, Piraccini BM, Strinchi C et al. Onychomycosis due to *Scopulariopsis brevicaulis*: clinical features and response to systemic antifungals. Br J Dermatol. 1996; 135: 799-802.
15. Tosti A, Piraccini BM. Proximal subungual onychomycosis due to Aspergillus niger. Report of two cases. Br J Dermatol. 1998; 139: 152-169.
16. Tosti A, Baran R, Piraccini BM, Fanti PA. Endonyx onychomycosis: a new modality of nail invasion by dermatophytic fungi. Acta Dermatovener. 1999; 79: 52-53.
17. Coleman R, Hay RJ. Chronic mucocutaneous candidosis associated with hypothyroidism: a distinct syndrome? Br J Dermatol. 1997; 136: 24-29.

Onychomycosis is so frequently encountered in daily practice that any nail dystrophy, especially one occurring in isolation, may be wrongly diagnosed. In addition, some entirely different dermatoses may cause similar nail alterations. This is due to the fact that the nail apparatus has a limited repertoire of reaction patterns and the nail plate covers and hides the very structures involved in the pathological process.

Some examples will be given [1, 2]:

● Distal lateral subungual onychomycosis with subungual hyperkeratosis.

This can be mimicked by several inflammatory nail conditions, characterized by their protracted and recalcitrant courses.

Psoriasis (Fig 4.1) is the skin disease that most often produces nail changes and can mimic onychomycosis even histologically (see p. 39), especially in the HIV-positive patient.

Subungual keratosis can be isolated or associated with onycholysis, leuconychia and distal splinter haemorrhages. As distortion and dystrophy of the nail plate may be seen in both onychomycosis and psoriasis, it may be impossible to diagnose psoriasis restricted to the nails on clinical grounds alone unless there is extensive pitting and/or the oil drop sign.

Psoriatic nails are said to be more susceptible to fungal infection (see ref. 49 on page 9).

Skin changes and nail features in **Reiter's syndrome** may be indistinguishable from those of patients with psoriasis. However, a brownish-red hue of the nail bed lesions may suggest this condition.

Pityriasis rubra pilaris (Fig 4.2).
In adult acute onset type I pityriasis rubra pilaris nail involvement usually presents as distal subungual hyperkeratosis with moderate thickening of the nail bed, splinter haemorrhages and longitudinal ridging.

Norwegian scabies (Fig 4.3)
The hyperkeratotic lesions are accompanied by large, psoriasis-like accumulations of scales under the nails and may resemble onychomycosis due to *T. rubrum* (Fig 4.4). The mites survive in these dystrophic nails and later colonize the skin, first around the nail plates. From there, they extend proximally. This type of scabies is most often seen in the old and infirm, the mentally defective, AIDS patients and during immunosuppression.

Fig 4.1
Psoriasis

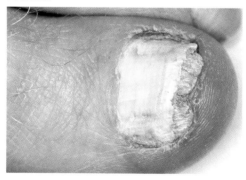

Fig 4.2
Pityriasis rubra pilaris

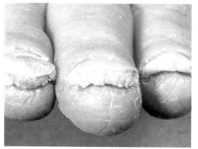
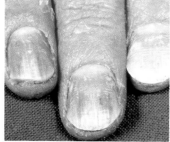

Courtesy R. Caputo (Milano)

Fig 4.3
Norwegian scabies

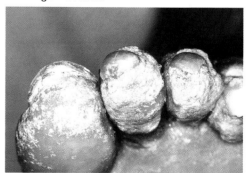

Fig 4.4
Chronic dermatophytic disease due to
T. rubrum

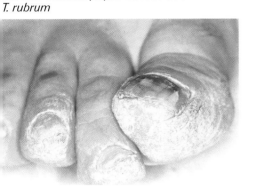

Fig 4.7
Chronic dermatitis

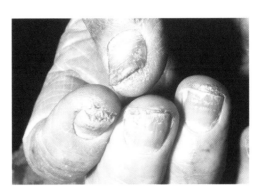

Fig 4.5
Darier's disease

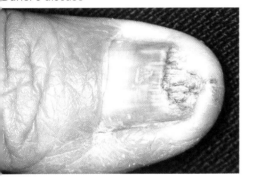

Darier's disease (Fig 4.5)
In typical cases the nails have longitudinal subungual pink or white streaks or both, and distal wedge-shaped subungual keratoses.

Lichen planus (Fig 4.6)
Usually there are a progressive thinning and fluting of the nail and marked subungual hyperkeratosis may lift the nail plate. It may therefore be associated with onycholysis which can sometimes be seen in isolation.

Chronic dermatitis (Fig 4.7).
The cause of nail changes is obvious when the eczema has a periungual distribution. It may be difficult to recognize in atopic dermatitis, discoid eczema etc.. The modifications of the nail result from disturbances of the matrix. These may present as thickening, pitting and transverse ridging sometimes leading to shedding of the nail.

Fig 4.6
Lichen planus

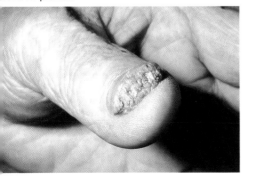

Clinical differential diagnosis

Fig 4.8
Actinic reticuloid erythroderma

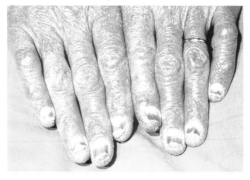

Erythroderma (Fig 4.8).
In chronic erythroderma due to Sézary's syndrome, for example, nail changes are similar to those found in patients with type I pityriasis rubra pilaris.

Pachyonychia congenita (Fig 4.9)
This is a hereditary ectodermal dysplasia with thickening of the nails which become yellow-brown tubular, hard and barrel-shaped. They project upward at their free edge while the subungual tissue is filled with keratotic material. The nail dystrophy appears usually within the first 6 months of life but later occurrence has been reported. Paronychia and onycholysis are common as well as recurrent shedding of the nail. Secondary *Candida* infection may occur.

Acrokeratosis paraneoplastica
(Bazex syndrome) (Fig 4.10)
It occurs in association with malignancy of the upper respiratory or digestive tract. In severe forms, the free edge is raised by subungual hyperkeratosis. The lesions resemble advanced psoriatic nail dystrophy and may progress to complete loss of the diseased nails.

Fig 4.9
Familial pachyonychia congenita

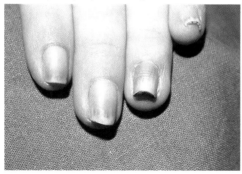

Courtesy G. Moulin (Lyon)

Fig 4.10
Acrokeratosis paraneoplastica

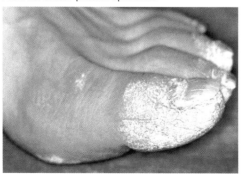

● Distal lateral subungual onychomycosis with onycholysis

Onycholysis can appear in many different conditions either dermatological such as psoriasis (Fig 4.11), lichen planus (Fig 4.12) and subungual tumours or systemic, including thyroid disease, yellow nail syndrome (Fig 4.13), etc. and may be produced by many medications.

In fingernails, primary onycholysis is more frequently associated with secondary invasion by *Candida* and/or *Pseudomonas*. It should be differentiated from nail plate-nail bed separation due to over zealous cleaning with an orange stick, for example.

Traumatic onycholysis of the toenails may present differently to that of fingernails. The diagnosis is obvious when the nail plate–nail bed separation appears after strenuous exercise in new footwear. Occasionally, a blackish hue may be the only presentation and is often due to the second toe overriding the big toe which results in subungual haemorrhage (Fig 4.14). This is more common in women. Patients with certain forms of epidermolysis bullosa are more susceptible to onycholysis.

Fig 4.12
Lichen planus

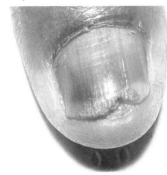

Courtesy S. Goettmann-Bonvallot (Paris)

Fig 4.13
Yellow nail syndrome

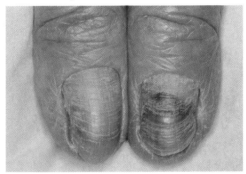

Fig 4.11
Psoriasis

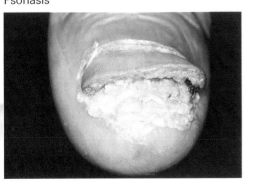

Fig 4.14
Repeated minor trauma

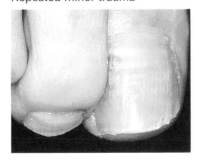 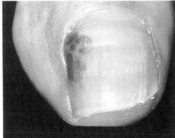

Clinical differential diagnosis

● **Superficial white onychomycosis**

Superficial friability can be produced by keratin granulations due to nail varnish or the base coat (Fig 4.15).

The psoriatic parakeratotic cells which usually disappear from the nail surface, leaving pitting, may be abnormally adherent to each other for a long period (Fig 4.16) – producing white superficial patches.

● **Proximal subungual onychomycosis**

This type of fungal infection, which may present with varied features (Fig 4.17), can be mimicked by :

– Longitudinal leuconychia in Darier's disease (Fig 4.18)

– Mild transverse leuconychia that may be monodactylous (single trauma or liquid nitrogen on the proximal nail fold), poly-dactylous (excessive manicure), or it may be due to repeated microtrauma to untrimmed toenails (Fig 4.19).

– Psoriatic transverse leuconychia (Fig 4.20) is often accompanied by pitting of the nail.

– Neurological disorders such as sympathetic reflex dystrophy, C4 spinal cord injury, etc.

– Arsenic (Mees' bands), thallium and, much more often, drug reactions due to cytotoxic drugs.

● **Proximal subungual onychomycosis with paronychia**

It can be mimicked by any cause of paronychia with subsequent nail dystrophy (Fig 4.21).

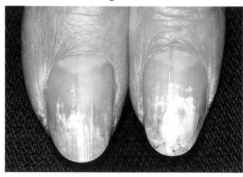

Fig 4.15
Nail varnish keratin granulations

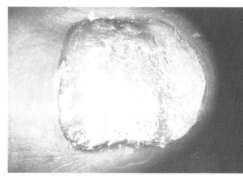

Fig 4.16
Psoriasis

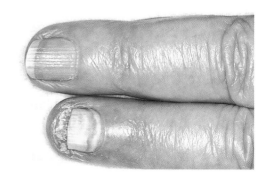

Fig 4.17
Proximal subungual onychomycosis due to *Fusarium*

Fig 4.18
Darier's disease

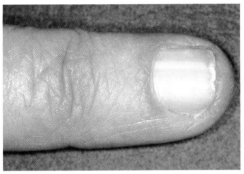

Fig 4.21
Leukaemic paronychia

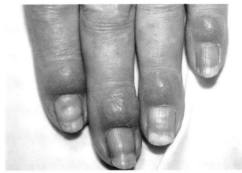

Courtesy H. A. Luscombe (USA)

Fig 4.19
Mechanical transverse leuconychia

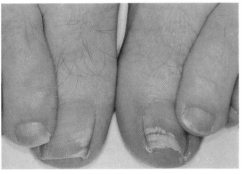

Fig 4.20
Transverse leuconychia due to psoriasis

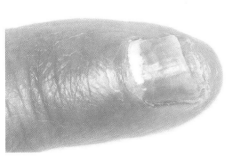

● **Fungal melanonychia** (Fig 4.22–24)

Haematoma, subungual tumours, foreign bodies, longitudinal melanonychia (Fig 4.23, 24) frictional melanonychia (Fig. 4.25) and even malignant melanoma (Fig 4.26–28) should be ruled out.

● **Bowen's disease and squamous cell carcinoma**

These malignant conditions may present as any of the above mentioned diseases (Fig 4.29).

Fig 4.22
Fungal melanonychia due to
Candida guilliermondii

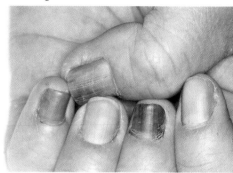

Fig 4.23
Fungal melanonychia due to
T. rubrum nigricans

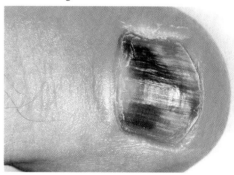

Fig 4.24
T. rubrum nigricans onychomycosis presenting as longitudinal melanonychia

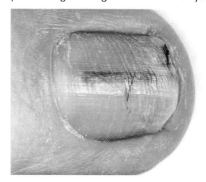

Fig 4.25
Frictional melanonychia

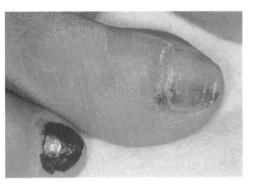

Fig 4.28
Malignant melanoma

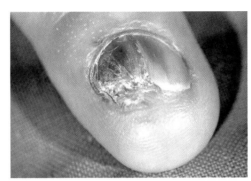

Fig 4.26
Acromelanoma

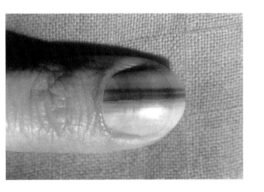

Fig 4.29
Bowen's disease

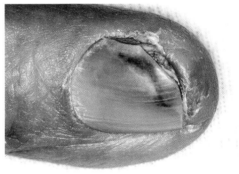

Fig 4.27
Malignant melanoma

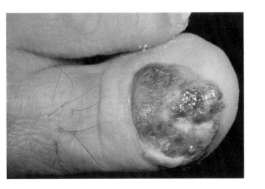

5 Mycological examination

The clinical patterns seen in fungal nail disease only provide a clue to the type of infection. Though certain types of nail involvement are characteristic of certain species, usually the clinical appearance caused by one species of fungus is indistinguishable from that caused by another. Therefore, the diagnosis of onychomycosis always requires laboratory confirmation. Mycological diagnosis of onychomycosis is based on detection of fungal elements in KOH or tetraethyl ammonium hydroxide preparations of the nail samples, histopathology and identification of the responsible fungus by culture [1-6]. This, however, may sometimes be difficult since fungi are not always isolated from nails due to their low number and viability. False negative mycological results are quite common especially when samples are taken from a distal nail clipping. A negative mycology does not therefore completely rule out onychomycosis since direct microscopy may be negative in up to 20% of cases and cultures may fail to isolate a fungus in up to 30% of cases. Recent treatment with topical antifungals may increase the chance of a false negative culture.

For this reason, when the clinical features strongly suggest onychomycosis, it is advisable to perform microscopic examination and culture more than once if initial investigations are negative. This is also recommended when the KOH preparation is positive and cultures are negative.

A glossary of terms is shown in Table 5.1.

Isolation of a fungus from a nail sample does not, on the other hand, necessarily indicate onychomycosis. Saprophytic fungi may colonize the nail and may be cultured from nail samples. Laboratory results should therefore always be carefully evaluated and it is very important to correlate the clinical with the mycological findings. The clinician must always bear in mind that some fungi such as yeasts and most non-dermatophytic moulds are nail saprophytes rather than pathogens.

A correct diagnosis of onychomycosis depends on several factors including accuracy of specimen collection, expertise of the laboratory and skill in the evaluation of the laboratory results.

5.1. The proper collection of samples: The "How" and "Where"

Correct collection of the specimen is essential in order to avoid false negative results as well as to eliminate contaminants (Fig 5.1). The site of specimen sampling depends on the clinical type of onychomycosis. It is always important to collect as much material as possible, since the nail may contain only a few fungal elements. Separate samples should be obtained from fingernails and toenails. Since toenail onychomycosis is frequently associated with tinea pedis, it is best to collect samples for mycology not only from the nails, but also from the soles. The same rule applies for the palms of patients with fingernail onychomycosis.

Table 5.1
Glossary

Conidia:	asexual spores
Dematiaceous:	brown-black pigmented fungus
Dermatophytes:	filamentous fungi specialized in the digestion of keratins
Floccose:	fluffy, cottony
Hyphae:	branching filaments formed by a chain of cells
Mycelium:	mass of hyphae
Moulds:	filamentous fungi
Phialide:	a conidiogenous cell that produces a succession of conidia from its tip
Spores:	reproductive cells
Yeasts:	unicellular budding fungi

● Distal subungual onychomycosis

Samples should be obtained from the nail bed and ventral nail plate. It is very important to try to collect material from the most proximal portion of the affected nail bed. This is the area most likely to contain viable fungi. The affected nail bed is exposed by removing the overlying onycholytic nail plate with a nail clipper; then appropriate material is taken by scraping the hyperkeratotic nail bed with a solid or disposable scalpel or a curette (Fig 5.2).

It is advisable, where possible, not to include the distal nail plate in the sample, since it frequently contains contaminants that may obscure the growth of pathogenic fungi.

● White superficial onychomycosis / Black superficial onychomycosis

Samples should be obtained from the friable areas of leuconychia (or melanonychia) of the superficial nail plate. Shallow shaving with a disposable scalpel or gently scraping the dorsum of the nail with a curette will provide specimens for microscopy and culture (Fig 5.3).

● Proximal subungual onychomycosis

Samples should be obtained from the intermediate nail plate. The affected nail plate is exposed by perforating the proximal nail with a disposable punch or an electric drill (Fig 5.4). The latter procedure offers the advantage of avoiding the necessity for anaesthesia and the risk of bleeding. Scales are then obtained by scraping the exposed nail plate with a disposable scalpel.

● Chronic paronychia

Samples can be taken from beneath the proximal nail fold by passing a disposable loop under the affected area of the fold, but the presence of *Candida* alone should not be interpreted as an indication that it is the only factor involved in causing the disease.

● Endonyx onychomycosis

Viable fungi are present throughout the whole thickness of the nail plate. Nail clippings can therefore be used for mycology.

Fig 5.1
Growth of contaminants from a distal nail clipping

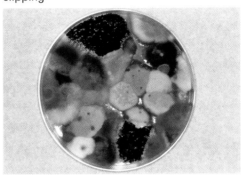

Fig 5.2
Collection of specimens from a nail affected by distal subungual onychomycosis.
Subungual scales are obtained with a curette after removal of the onycholytic nail plate

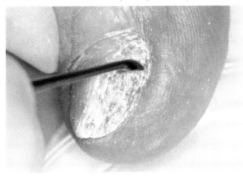

Fig 5.3
Collection of specimens from a nail affected by white superficial onychomycosis.
The leuconychial area is directly scraped with a curette

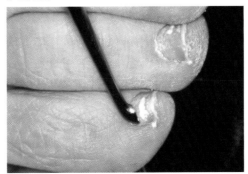

Mycological examination

5.2 Microscopic examination

After collection, specimens are placed in a Petri dish or in a dark envelope or mailing pack and sent to the laboratory. Immediate examination is not mandatory since fungi remain viable in nail specimens for several months.

Before examination, the nail material is divided into small fragments; half of the sample is usually used for direct microscopy and the other half for culture. Thick materials need to be pulverized; this can be achieved by crushing the nail specimens with a hammer or using a nail micronizer.

The nail material is placed on a glass slide with a drop of 20-30% KOH. After applying a coverslip, gently heating the slide in a Bunsen flame accelerates clearing the keratin with visualization of the fungal elements. The coverslip is then gently pushed down with a pencil to flatten the scales. Screening should be carried out as soon as possible to avoid deterioration of the specimen.

Using 20% KOH in a vehicle of 60% water and 40% DMSO provides a more rapid method of diagnosis of mycosis without heating, and the specimen lasts longer for re-examination.

Identification of fungi may be facilitated by adding a drop of Chlorazol Black E (Sigma), a counter stain specific for chitin to the KOH preparation. Only the fungal elements develop a greenish blue colour and Chlorazol Black E may help to differentiate these from artefacts. Alternatively the hyphae can be stained with a fluorochrome (calcofluor white) but this requires a fluorescence microscope. It is, however, a very accurate method of screening nails.

The microscope is set with the condenser in a low position and the diaphragm shut down in order to produce a dark background that contrasts with the light-refracting hyphae. The slide is first screened at low power (10 x objective). Details can be discerned using 40 x objective. Fungal hyphae appear as elongated branching, septate, light-refracting structures that pass across the horny cells (Fig 5.5). It is impossible to differentiate non viable from viable fungi. Fungal elements should be differentiated from artefacts including lipid vesicles, air bubbles,

Fig 5.4
Collection of specimens in a case of proximal subungual onychomycosis.
Scales are collected from the intermediate nail after perforation of the nail plate with a disposable punch

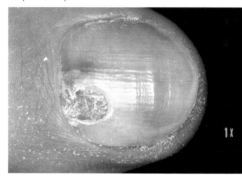

Fig 5.5
KOH preparation of a nail sample showing refractial branching hyphae

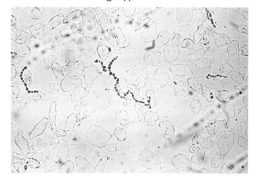

textile fibres and mosaic fungus. The latter is a common artefact caused by lipid deposition at the periphery of the host cells.

Microscopic examination can differentiate yeast cells from dermatophyte hyphae and other moulds, but species identification cannot be made from wet mounts. However, *Scopulariopsis brevicaulis* may be identified when thick-walled, pigmented lemon-shaped spores are seen (Fig 5.6), and *Scytalidium dimidiatum*, or *S. hyalinum* suspected by their narrow tortuous hyphae.

Since different causative organisms (Table 5.2) may require different therapies, reliable identification of the causal agent is important and this can only be made by culture.

5.3. Culture

Half of the specimen should be set up for culture even when microscopic examination is negative.

In order to grow both dermatophytes and non-dermatophytes it is always important to inoculate the material into two different media :

1. Sabouraud glucose-agar with 0.05% chloramphenicol that permits the growth of dermatophytes, non-dermatophytes and yeasts.

2. Sabouraud glucose-agar with 0.05% chloramphenicol and 0.4% cycloheximide (Actidione®), which allows the growth of dermatophytes, but inhibits the growth of yeasts and most non-dermatophytic moulds.

Inoculation is made using a sterile needle and 10 to 20 pieces of specimen are gently pushed into each medium. Cultures are incubated at 24–28°C. Non-dermatophytic moulds grow faster than dermatophytes and produce well formed colonies within 1 week. Colonies of most dermatophytes are usually completely differentiated in 2 weeks. A negative result is the absence of growth after 3–6 weeks. All plates should be kept for a minimum of 2 weeks in case mould or yeast growth obscures that of a dermatophyte.

Identification of the fungi is based on growth rate and the macroscopic and microscopic appearance of the colony. For this purpose, a small portion of the colony is selected by pressing a strip of Sellotape onto the surface of the culture. The tape is then placed on a slide and stained with lactophenol cotton blue. Alternatively, pieces of colony can be teased out with a sterile needle.

Media containing a phenol red pH indicator that changes from yellow to red in the presence of dermatophytes are also available on the market (DTM) (Fig 5.7). These media contain antibiotics and cycloheximide to inhibit contaminant bacteria and fungi. However, some contaminants can still grow in the medium and produce a red discoloration that can be erroneously interpreted as a sign of dermatophyte growth. Although routine use of these media is not recommended, they can be helpful when laboratory facilities are not available.

Fig 5.6
KOH preparation of a *Scopulariopsis brevicaulis* nail infection.
Elongated branching hyphae together with lemon-shaped conidia characteristic of this fungus are shown

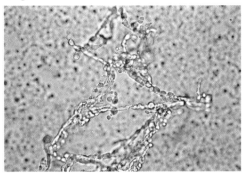

Fig 5.7
Proof of growth of dermatophytes (DTM).
In case of growth the medium changes its colour to red

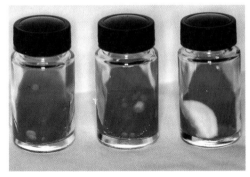

Mycological examination

Table 5.2
Causative organisms of onychomycosis

	Common	Uncommon
Dermatophytes	*T. rubrum* *T. mentagrophytes var. interdigitale*	*Epidermophyton floccosun* *T. soudanense* *T. violaceum* *T. mentagrophytes var. mentagrophytes* *M. canis* *T. tonsurans* *T. erinacei* *T. equinum* *M. gypseum*
Moulds	*Scopulariopsis brevicaulis* *Fusarium* spp.	*Acremonium* spp. *Aspergillus* spp. *Scytalidium* spp. *Onychocola canadensis* *Chaetomium globosum* *Paecilomyces* spp.
Yeasts		*Candida albicans* *Candida parapsilosis*

Dermatophytes

T. rubrum – Within 2 weeks *T. rubrum* forms dome-shaped floccose white colonies with a well defined dark red-brown to yellow reverse (Fig 5.8, 5.9).

Lactophenol cotton blue mounts of the colonies show sparse club-shaped microconidia along the sides of the hyphae.

T. mentagrophytes var. **interdigitale** – Within 2 weeks *T. interdigitale* forms powdery white colonies with a cream centre and a pale to dark-brown reverse (Fig 5.10).

Lactophenol cotton blue mounts of the colonies reveal abundant microconidia along the sides and at the ends of branched hyphae (Fig 5.11). Characteristic spiral hyphae may be present.

Fig 5.8
Trichophyton rubrum.
Macroscopic appearance of the colony and its reverse (5.9) two weeks after inoculation

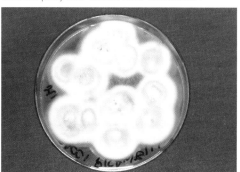

Fig 5.9

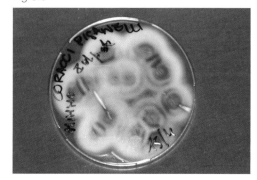

Non-dermatophytic moulds

Non-dermatophytic moulds are widespread in the environment as soil and plant saprophytes, and can frequently be found in the nails as contaminants. Isolating a non-dermatophyte mould from nail material does not necessarily have any pathological significance and the results of cultures should always be correlated with the nail signs. In particular, non-dermato-phytic moulds are commonly isolated from toenails affected by traumatic onycholysis, onychogryphosis and pachyonychia, where they are present as saprophytes.

Laboratory diagnosis of non-dermatophyte mould onychomycosis requires the following criteria [7]:

- presence of hyphae in the KOH preparation; sometimes these are irregular in shape or are pigmented.

- growth of the fungus in at least five inocula on the same plate.

- isolation of the same mould from three consecutive nail samples.

Scopulariopsis brevicaulis – *Scopulariopsis brevicaulis* grows in both media with and without cycloheximide. Within 1 week it forms brown colonies with powdery surfaces and pale brown reverse (Fig 5.12).

Lactophenol cotton blue mounts of the colonies reveal numerous branched conidio-phores with chains of lemon-shaped conidia.

Fusarium spp. – Growth of *Fusarium* spp. requires cycloheximide-free medium. Within a week *Fusarium* spp. produce flat colonies which are pale pink or brownish in colour (Fig 5.13).

Culture mounts in lactophenol cotton blue show numerous sickle-shaped macroconidia and elliptical and oval microconidia. These arise from short phialidic cells in colonies of *Fusarium oxysporum,* or long phialidic cells in colonies of *Fusarium solani.*

Aspergillus spp. – Growth of *Aspergillus* spp. requires cycloheximide-free medium. The macroscopic appearance of the colonies varies among the different species.

Lactophenol cotton blue mounts of the colonies are diagnostic due to the typical vesiculate heads, and conidial chains.

Fig 5.10
Trichophyton interdigitale.
Macroscopic appearance of the colony
2 weeks after inoculation

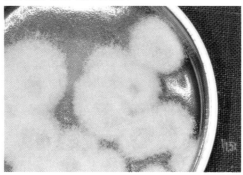

Fig 5.11
Lactophenol cotton blue mount of a colony of *Trichophyton interdigitale* .
Abundant round microconidia along the sides and at the ends of branched hyphae are shown

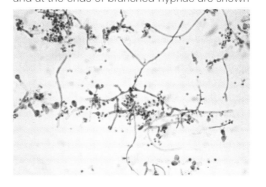

Fig 5.12
Scopulariopsis brevicaulis.
Macroscopic appearance of the colony
2 weeks after inoculation

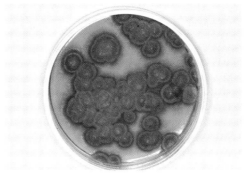

Mycological examination

Acremonium spp. – *Acremonium* spp. grow in media both with and without cycloheximide. In cycloheximide-free medium *Acremonium* forms white-pink velvety colonies within 1 week.

Lactophenol cotton blue mounts of the colonies reveal elliptical conidia grouped at the tips of long phialides. They can be confused with *Fusarium* spp.

Scytalidium spp. – In cycloheximide-free medium, *Scytalidium* spp. produce fast growing colonies with an abundant aerial mycelium that, in some cultures, fills a Petri dish within a few days. Others are slower. Colonies of *Scytalidium dimidiatum* are initially white and become black or dark brown in a few days, while colonies of *Scytalidium hyalinum* remain white or creamy in colour.

Lactophenol cotton blue mounts of the colonies reveal the chains of arthrospores, which are brown-walled in the colonies of *Scytalidium dimidiatum*.

5.4. Histopathological examination

Unna was the first to give a detailed histopathological description of favus infected nails [8]. Particular histopathological patterns of infection were described later [9–12]. Almost all mycologists and most dermatologists would agree that direct microscopy of KOH-cleared specimens and mycological cultures are the gold standard for the diagnosis of skin and nail mycoses. However, histopathology has its undoubted advantages and is sometimes clearly superior to the routine mycological diagnostic procedures. The result of histopathological examinations is much faster than culture – usually 3 days versus 3 weeks – and histopathology is more often positive than cultures [13–18]. It also shows whether there are hyphae and/or spores, whether the fungal organisms grow as invasive filamentous pathogens in the nail plate and/or in the subungual hyperkeratosis, and how the nail is damaged by the pathogenic fungi [13, 19]. It is often the only means to differentiate ungual psoriasis from onychomycosis.

Histopathology can be performed on nail plate material preferably containing as much subungual debris as possible and from nail

Fig 5.13
Fusarium solani.
Macroscopic appearence of the colony 1 week after inoculation

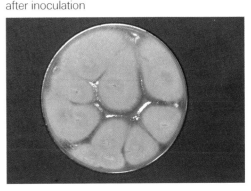

biopsies. Routinely, PAS staining is sufficient for the diagnosis, confirmation or exclusion of onychomycosis in more than 90 % of cases. Enrichment of the specimen using the KONCPA technique (**KO**H treated **N**ail **C**lippings stained with **PA**S) may further enhance the sensitivity of histopathology [20]. Additional stains like Grocott's and Gridley's may be used; however, they very rarely give a positive result when PAS was negative. Fluorochromation using a blancophore is even more specific; this fluorescent dye specifically stains fungal cell walls because of their chitin content [21]. The technicians require some experience to produce good sections [18, 21, 22].

Nail plate material can be obtained by clipping as much of the distal nail plate as possible. This is sufficient in the case of distal-lateral subungual onychomycosis. For superficial white onychomycosis, a layer of the dorsal surface of the nail plate may be cut tangentially from the nail using a #23 or #15 scalpel. Proximal white subungual onychomycosis very often demonstrates proximal onycholysis, thus allowing the physician to take a punch biopsy from the nail plate without prior anaesthesia. The little nail disc may be cut into two halves, one for histopathology, the other one for mycological culture.

Nail biopsies are not commonly required to make the diagnosis of distal subungual onychomycosis, but may be the only means to differentiate onychomycosis from nail psoriasis, lichen planus, alopecia areata, nail eczema, and other inflammatory nail disorders. Usually, a lateral longitudinal nail biopsy is taken yielding a 2 mm wide block of tissue containing the entire length of the nail plate with overlying proximal nail fold, underlying matrix, nail bed, hyponychium and adjacent skin of the tip of the digit.

Histopathology of nail plate specimens varies according to the clinical type of onychomycosis, the severity of the nail changes and the abundance of fungi in and under the nail. As for mycological cultures, subungual keratinous debris mostly contains more fungal elements than the plate itself (Fig 5.14). The histopathology of nail biopsies confirms the findings in nail clippings, but also gives information about the involvement of the soft ungual tissues that are responsible for nail growth, attachment to the nail bed and the nail's appearance.

Distal lateral subungual onychomycosis.
Fungal hyphae are usually found in the nail plate undersurface. Fine filaments are arranged in a longitudinal direction, often remarkably parallel which is a sign of a hitherto undisturbed nail growth. Depending on the severity, they may be seen as slender, septate hyphae in a compact nail plate or as thick, septate elements showing shorter and longer intersections as well as relatively large round spores. The latter are seen to have a basophilic content in H&E stains and are probably dermatophyte arthrospores (Fig 5.15). Subungual keratinous material may adhere to the nail plate and contain very large amounts of spores and short thick hyphae. They are able to invade the nail plate causing splits as well as vertical and branching defects in the deep nail plate layers. Quite often, the thick subungual hyperkeratosis appears papillomatous and contains large globules of dried serum (Fig. 5.14) as well as intracorneal neutrophils morphologically indistinguishable from Munro's microabscesses. Fungal filaments are also seen in close vicinity to the serum although dermatophytes are presumed not to grow in the presence of serum. Subungual debris often contains huge numbers of large, thick-walled, polyhedral spores between horny cells; they may however germinate and short thick filaments penetrate the nail plate.
The clinical phenomenon of yellow longitudinal streak which is often seen in dermatophytic toenail infections shows abundant large, extremely thick-walled spores and short

Fig 5.14a
Nail clippings from distal subungual onychomycosis.
Undersurface of nail plate and subungual hyperkeratosis containing abundant slender hyphae of *Trichophyton rubrum*. PAS, magnification 250 x

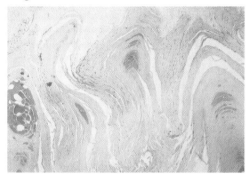

Fig 5.14b
Undersurface of nail plate containing fungal filaments and spores.
Blancophore fluorochromation, magnification 250 x

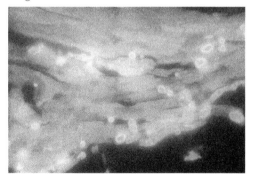

filaments compressed in a tube-like space formed by the overlying nail plate and subungual keratin.

Longitudinal nail biopsies show essentially the same type of alteration though to a very variable degree. The nail bed develops subungual hyperkeratosis that initially covers the distal portion of the nail bed but progresses proximally toward the matrix. It contains abundant hyphae, quite often large amounts of serum and often also pycnotic neutrophils and a few lymphocytes. The neutrophils may form typical intracorneal spongiform abscesses which, however, are usually situated within predominantly orthokeratotic hyperkeratoses. The more severe the onychomycosis the more proximally these changes will have advanced. The nail plate itself is only invaded in its lower layers. The fungi are seen to lie in a longitudinal parallel arrangement. The nail bed epithelium may exhibit considerable spongiosis with lymphocytic exocytosis but only few intermingled neutrophils. There may be a dense mononuclear inflammatory infiltrate in the upper dermis with some accentuation perivascularly. When distal subungual onychomycosis secondarily progresses to total dystrophic onychomycosis, nail bed and matrix alterations become more pronounced. The epithelium may become papillomatous, heavily oedematous and infiltrated with neutrophils and/or lymphocytes. Pseudobullous subepithelial oedema may develop. The distal nail plate breaks away but the proximal third under the proximal nail fold usually remains more or less intact.

Superficial white onychomycosis.
The same alterations are seen in nail biopsies as in clippings or shave biopsies. Either chains of regularly sized small spores occur in splits of the nail plate surface or short hyphae and spores have invaded the surface layers. There is no inflammatory infiltrate in the nail bed beneath the fungal invasion (Fig. 5.16).

Fig 5.15 b
Branched septate hyphae are seen in the nail plate above the spores.
PAS, magnification 1000 x

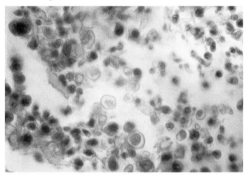

Fig 5.15 c
Large spores are situated in a nail plate defect.
PAS, magnification 1000 x

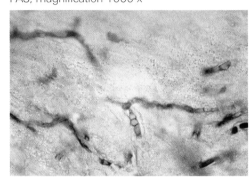

Fig 5.15 a
Huge masses of spores and few short hyphae are seen in deep nail plate layers.
Undersurface of nail plate with fungi and serum globules. PAS, magnification 100 x

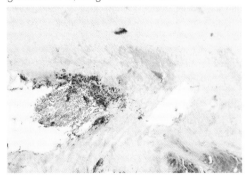

Fig 5.16
Superficial white onychomycosis.
PAS, magnification 400 x

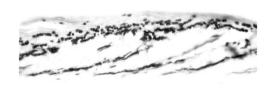

Endonyx onychomycosis. This is usually due to *T. soudanense* infection. Large amounts of hyphae are seen in the nail plate virtually without involvement of the nail bed. Inflammatory changes are practically absent (Fig.5.17) [23].

Proximal white subungual onychomycosis. Punched nail plate usually shows a compact nail plate without inflammatory cells. The entire thickness of the plate may be invaded by large amounts of fungal filaments that are arranged longitudinally and in a parallel manner. Almost total nail plate invasion was also seen in a case of *Candida albicans* proximal onychomycosis in a new-born (unpublished observation). Nail biopsies show some fungal filaments in the stratum corneum of the undersurface of the proximal nail fold. From here, fungi may also invade the nail plate surface (Fig 5.18) which may give rise to the picture of superficial white onychomycosis growing out from under the nail fold. There is only a sparse inflammatory reaction to the fungal infection of the eponychium. The pathogens slowly progress toward the proximal tip of the matrix. When the latter is reached the relatively fast growing matrix cells differentiating into onychocytes, will incorporate the fungi and transport them distally while the nail plate grows out. Part of the fungi further progress along the matrix-nail plate junction in a distal direction toward the nail bed. All along the matrix, fungal elements are continuously included in the growing nail plate and thus transported away from the epithelium. This is the reason for amazingly little inflammatory response to the infection in the matrix area, but it also explains why in this particular form of nail infection, fungi are found in all layers of the nail plate. When the fungi arrive at the nail bed they induce a reaction similar to that seen in distal subungual onychomycosis with nail bed hyperkeratosis and inflammation. Proximal subungual onychomycosis due to *Candida albicans* may also occur in chronic mucocutaneous candidosis [24].

Total dystrophic onychomycosis. Only small nail plate fragments are left or irregular hyperkeratoses overlie the nail field. Nail plate remnants with keratotic debris show variable amounts of fungal elements that are haphazardly arranged. There are also inflammatory cells and serum inclusions. Particularly in chronic mucocutaneous candidosis, the orderly nail structure is completely lost. The proximal

Fig 5.17
Endonyx onychomycosis.
PAS, magnification 250 x

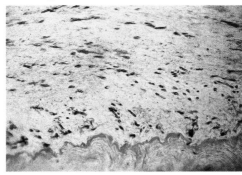

Fig 5.18
Proximal subungual onychomycosis
exhibiting marked hyperkeratosis (HK) of
the ventral surface of the proximal nail fold (NF)
and fungal filaments in the nail plate (NP)
matrix (M). Grocott, magnification 100 x

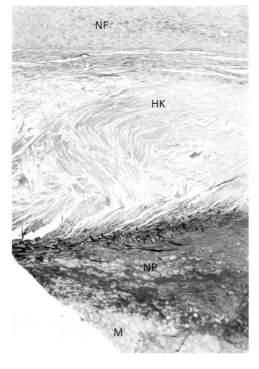

Mycological examination

Fig 5.19a
Total dystrophic onychomycosis
secondary to distal subungual dermatophyte
infection. PAS, magnification 100 x

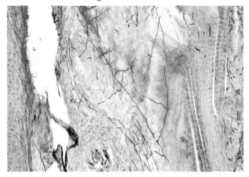

Fig 5.19b
Primary total dystrophic onychomycosis
in a patient with chronic mucocutaneous
candidosis. Grocott, magnification 250 x

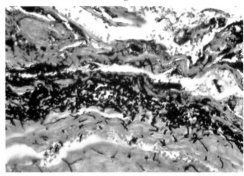

nail fold has receded to form a short rim of tissue. Matrix and nail bed are papillomatous and
hyperkeratotic with alternating hypergranulosis.
Fungal filaments and spores irregularly penetrate the hyperkeratoses (Fig. 5.19). Electron
microscopy shows *Candida* spores and germ
tubes. The matrix and nail bed epithelia respond
with marked keratohyalin granule production
and composite keratohyalin granules are
abundant. Exocytosis of lymphocytes is evident
with many of them exhibiting convoluted
nuclei [25].

Nail destruction by fungi

Histopathological examination of nail material
also allows the degree of nail dystrophy due to
fungal invasion to be studied. A few spores
scattered in splits of subungual keratin are
probably just commensals. Large amounts of
fungal organisms, whether filaments or spores,
have to be considered pathogens. Commonly
spores and short thick hyphae are seen to lie in
spaces of nail or subungual keratin. They often
penetrate into the nail from beneath. The nail
keratin next to the holes formed by the fungi
often stains more eosinophilic indicating
chemical digestion. Very large amounts of fungi
penetrating the entire thickness of the nail plate
also reduce the mechanical resistance of the
plate (Fig. 5.19).

Determination of fungi

Histopathology can distinguish between
commensals and pathogens, however, it
cannot determine the fungal species. Long
slender hyphae are usually dermatophytes, but

Scytalidium dimidiatum and *S. hyalinum* look
the same. Short, branched, thick filaments are
probably non-dermatophyte moulds. Dermatophytes can form huge amounts of thick-walled
spores also resembling non-dermatophyte
moulds. *Scopulariopsis brevicaulis* usually forms
large polygonal spores. *Candida albicans* may
be identified by spores that form germ tubes.

Immunohistochemistry using antibodies
against pathogenetically relevant fungi as well
as flow cytometry have been used to identify
the pathogens of onychomycosis [26]. However, it has to be stressed that up to now, only
mycological cultures are able to reliably identify
the fungal pathogen.

Differential diagnosis

Psoriasis and onychomycosis can be
indistinguishable on clinical and sometimes
even on histological grounds. They share the
same features although to different degrees.
Psoriasis of the nail has prominent parakeratosis, subungual intracorneal leucocytes,
sometimes spongiform pustules, and the
characteristic pits. The latter may be seen to
contain parakeratosis when the pit is on the nail
plate surface still under the proximal nail fold.
Onychomycosis usually shows alternating
orthokeratosis and parakeratosis, abundant
neutrophils and Munro's microabscesses, but
no pits (Table 5.3) [27]. The value of histopathology both for the rapid diagnosis as well as
for the differentiation from ungual psoriasis has
recently been confirmed by three more groups
[28–30].

Table 5.3

Histopathological differentiation of onychomycosis and ungual psoriasis

Feature	Onychomycosis	Psoriasis
Fungal elements	usually abundant	only occur in secondary "onycho-mycotization" or as saprophytes
Pits with parakeratosis	absent	rarely seen in sections but very characteristic
Intracorneal leucocytes and Munro's microabscesses	very frequent	very frequent
Spongiform pustules	rare	common, particularly in pustular psoriasis
Spongiosis	common	common
Exocytosis	leucocytes, few lymphocytes	leucocytes, few lymphocytes

References

1. Midgley G, Moore MK, Cook JC et al. Mycology of nail disorders. J Am Acad Dermatol. 1994; 31 : 568–574.
2. Elewski BE. Clinical pearl: diagnosis of onychomycosis. J Am Acad Dermatol. 1995; 32 : 500–501.
3. Clayton Y & Midgley G. Medical Mycology. Gower Medical Publishing, 1985, London .
4. Evans EGV, Richardson MD. Medical mycology: a medical approach. IRL Press, Oxford, 1989.
5. Campbell CK, Johnson EM, Philpot CM, Warnock DW. Identification of pathogenic fungi. Public Health Laboratory Service, London, 1996.
6. Lasagni A. Atlante di micologia. UTET Periodici Scientifici, Milano, 1996.
7. English MP. Nails and fungi. Br J Dermatol. 1976; 94 : 697–701.
8. Unna PG. The Histopathology of the Diseases of the Skin. Edinburgh: W F Clay; 1896: 342
9. Alkiewicz J. Transverse net in the diagnosis of onychomycosis. Arch Dermatol 1948; 58:385–389
10. Sagher F. Histologic examinations of fungous infections of the nails. J Invest Dermatol 1948; 11:337–357
11. Stühmer A. Subunguale Epidermophytie, Trichophytie und Favus. Eine bisher nicht bekannte Form von Nagelmykosen. Arch Dermatol Syph 1952; 193:527–536

12. Tosti A. Endonyx onychomycosis due to Trichophyton soudanense. Submitted.
13. Haneke E. Nail biopsies in onychomycosis. Mykosen 1985; 28:473
14. Bojanovsky A. Zur Bewertung des histologischen Nachweises von Onychomykosen. Castellania 1975; 3:169–171
15. Hauck H. Histologische Untersuchungen bei Nagelmykosen. 12th Scient Meet German Soc Mycol, Baden/Vienna, 1975, Book of Abstr p. 7
16. Achten G, Wanet-Rouard J. Onychomycoses in the laboratory. Mykosen 1978; Suppl 1:125–127
17. Scher RK, Ackerman AB. Subtle clues to diagnosis from biopsies of nails. The value of nail biopsy for demonstrating fungi not demonstrable by microbiologic techniques. Am J Dermatopathol 1980; 2:55–57
18. Haneke E. Bedeutung der Nagelhistologie für die Diagnostik und Therapie der Onychomykosen. Ärztl Kosmetol 1988; 18:248–254
19. Haneke E. Differential diagnosis of mycotic nail diseases. In Hay JR, ed. Advances in Topical Antifungal Therapy. Berlin Heidelberg New York: Springer, 1986:94
20. Liu HN, Lee DD, Wong CK. KONCPA: a new method for diagnosing tinea unguium. Dermatology 1993; 187:166–168
21. Haneke E. Fungal infections of the nail. Sem Dermatol 1991; 10: 41–53
22. Mondragon G. A method for processing specimens of nails. Dermatopathol Pract Concept 1996; 2:41–42

23. Baran R, Hay RJ, Tosti A, Haneke E. A new classification of onychomycoses. Br J Dermatol 1998; 139: 567–571
24. Baran R. Proximal subungual candida onychomycosis. An unusual manifestation of chronic mucocutaneous candidosis. Br J Dermatol 1997; 137:286–288
25. Haneke E. The nails in chronic mucocutaneous candidosis. Abstr, 15th Ann Meet Soc Cut Ultrastruct Res, Nice 1988
26. Piérard GE, Arrese JE, Pierre S, Bertrand C, Corcuff P, Levèque JL, Piérard-Franchimont C. Diagnostic microscopique des onychomycoses. Ann Dermatol Vénérérol 1994; 121:25–29
27. Haneke E. Onychomycosis and psoriasis restricted to the nails – distinguishable? 50th Ann Meeting Am Acad Dermatol, Dallas TX, Dec 7–12, 1991
28. Baral J, Fusco F, Kahn H, Ramsinghani R, Phelps RG. The use of nail clippings for detecting fungi in nail plates. Dermatopathol Pract Concept 1996; 2:266–268
29. Mehregan DA, Mehregan DR, Rinker A. Onychomycosis. Cutis 1997; 59: 247–248
30. Machler BC, Kirsner RS, Elgart GW. Routine histologic examination for the diagnosis of onychomycosis: An evaluation of sensitivity and specificity. Cutis 1998; 61: 217–219

The desired end points in the treatment of onychomycosis are both a negative mycology and a normal looking nail. Consequently, the goals are twofold:

1. mycological cure
2. clinical recovery of the nail

Fig 6.1
Linear nail growth in fingernails

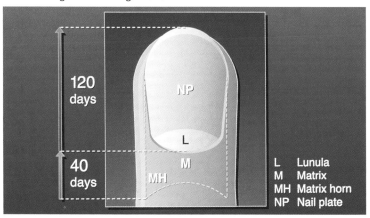

Fig 6.2
Linear nail growth in toenails

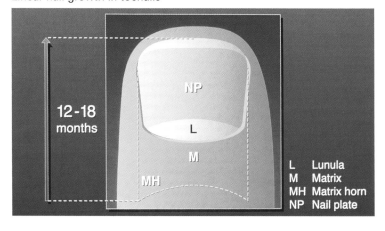

Mycological cure

Eradication of the fungus is confirmed by KOH examination (see p. 30) and culture (see p. 31). In many treatment studies, entry criteria require that all patients have a positive culture and KOH, however the reproducibility of these assesssments and their consistency through the study is poor, for as many as one third of those with a negative culture may have had false negative results on retesting [1]. Therefore, when sampling for microscopy and culture during treatment, it is quite common that there are discrepancies between KOH and culture results for the following reasons : since the killing rate of the fungi is far higher than the disappearance of the hyphae at the distal end of the nail plate which is dependent on the nail growth rate, direct microscopy may still be positive when cultures are negative. In addition, standard microscopy cannot distinguish living from dead filaments; therefore, some authors suggest that it cannot be used to measure the response of nails to antifungal drugs [2]. However, complete absence of fungal hyphae in KOH examination is a definite proof for the absence of a fungal infection.

Since the goal for the treatment of onychomycosis is complete cure, this should be defined according to two important but sometimes neglected parameters, the linear nail growth and the possible preexisting condition of the nail plate, discussed further on.

The fingernails grow 0.1 mm daily and the toenails at half to one-third this rate (Fig 6.1, 2). As the rate of linear nail growth decreases by 0.5% per year [3], elderly patients, who have a relatively slow linear nail growth rate, are therefore particularly susceptible to fungal infection [4]. Nail growth is also affected by other physiological and environmental factors as gender, right/left handedness, and environmental temperature as well as by systemic and cutaneous disease [5].

Patients with DLSO often have a decreased growth rate of the nail compared with that of controls. Consequently, the growth rate of the nail plate should be considered in the pathogenesis of onychomycosis [6]. Nevertheless, a recent investigation has questioned the relationship between slow linear nail growth rate and onychomycosis [7]. The mean rate of linear nail growth in 30 patients previously affected by onychomycosis was not significantly different to that of the control patients. Therefore, this study did not support the view that slow growth of the nail was a predisposing cause for fungal nail disease. Other factors such as local abnormality of the nails, which are more common in older patients, may be responsible for the increased incidence of onychomycosis in this group [8]. However irrespective of the predisposing factors for onychomycosis, it may be tempting to use anti-fungals (or other drugs) likely to increase the rate of the linear nail growth since the rapid achievement of a normal nail plate is desirable.

Clearance of the nail plate

Clearance of the nail plate is defined either by:

a) **clinical cure** with 100% clearance of signs, or

b) **clinical success,** with a residual affected nail area smaller than 10%. This corresponds to residual onychomycosis but might include previous nail dystrophy of unknown aetiology.

Chronic trauma implies repeated minor injury often unnoticed by the patient. A history of nail trauma as a cause of nail dystrophy can therefore be difficult to elicit and can be an aggravating factor in treatment. Repeated microtrauma to the toenail would be of little importance were it not for the shoes of the fashion-conscious woman and its significance for the sport's enthusiast and in the elderly where impaired ambulation may play a prominent role [9].

Repeated microtrauma is thought to play a major role in eliciting fungal invasion, especially mould onychomycosis. It also produces a wide range of nail abnormalities which will remain after completion of the treatment of onychomycosis despite mycological cure, since the fungal infection has affected a previously damaged nail.

It follows from the statements expressed above about the accuracy of the criteria commonly used to assess recovery after drug therapy, mycological and clinical cure, that although these methods are simple and effective in many instances, those interpreting the results of clinical trials must be aware of these potential pitfalls in assessment of response.

Goals for the treatment of onychomycosis

Clinical measurement and assessment of responses

It has been said that "the methodology" used for the assessment of response is a "muddle, illogical in almost all its aspects" [2].

To evaluate the effects of treatment, the junction between normal and diseased nail bed can be marked by cutting a wedge mark on the surface of the nail (Fig 6.3,4). This notch followed over timed intervals moves distally as the nail grows; the junction of infected and uninfected nail bed coincide if the treatment is effective [10]. However, this method may be difficult to carry out accurately in toenails where irregular lacunae within the nail plate due to onychomycosis may remain and delay recovery.

To assess the speed and extent of the response Hay et al. [11] used area instead of length, to calculate a % rate of nail restitution. The difficulty with area is that, unlike length, change is non-linear because the proximal nail is variously concealed by the folds and does not correspond to the nail area beneath. This is not solved by measuring changes in the area of involved nail (instead of unaffected nail) since this area can be altered by nail clipping [2].

Shuster has devised a new method [2] for measuring nail response totally independent of degree of involvement of the nail and the rate of nail growth. The principle is as follows: in the common distal onychomycosis, disease grows proximally: if the causal fungi were to die suddenly, the outward movement of disease could be no faster than the growth rate of nail and associated subungual keratin. In this system the measure of therapeutic efficacy is a dimensionless number, the ratio of the actual rate of outward movement of disease to the maximal possible rate which is the underlying rate of outward growth of nail:

$$\frac{\text{disease movement}}{\text{nail growth}}$$

a ratio in mm/mm for length, or mm^2/mm^2 for area.

At present this scheme is not widely used but it seems to underscore the unsatisfactory nature of current methods of assessment of nail recovery.

Fig 6.3
Assessment of drug effectiveness

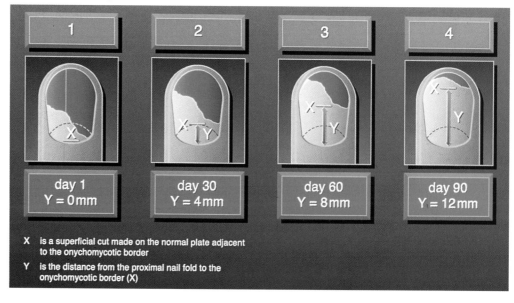

1	2	3	4
day 1 Y = 0mm	day 30 Y = 4mm	day 60 Y = 8mm	day 90 Y = 12mm

X is a superficial cut made on the normal plate adjacent to the onychomycotic border

Y is the distance from the proximal nail fold to the onychomycotic border (X)

Fig 6.4
Assessment of drug effectiveness

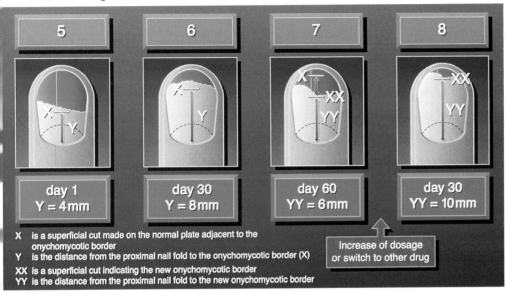

5	6	7	8
day 1 Y = 4 mm	day 30 Y = 8 mm	day 60 YY = 6 mm	day 30 YY = 10 mm

Increase of dosage
or switch to other drug

X   is a superficial cut made on the normal plate adjacent to the onychomycotic border
Y   is the distance from the proximal nail fold to the onychomycotic border (X)
XX is a superficial cut indicating the new onychomycotic border
YY is the distance from the proximal nail fold to the new onychomycotic border

References

1. Smith EB. Topical antifungal drugs in the treatment of tinea pedis, tinea cruris, and tinea corporis. J Am Acad Dermatol. 1993; 28: S24-S28.

2. Shuster S. Onychomycosis: Making sense of the assessment of antifungal drugs. Acta Dermatovener. 1998; 78: 1-4.

3. Orentreich N, Markofsky J, Volgelman JH. The effect of aging on the rate of linear nail growth. J Invest Dermatol. 1979; 73: 126-130.

4. English MP, Atkinson R. Onychomycosis in elderly chiropody patients. Br J Dermatol. 1974; 91: 67-72.

5. Dawber RPR, de Berker D, Baran R. Science of the nail apparatus in Baran R, Dawber RPR (eds) Diseases of the nails and their management. Blackwell Oxford, 1994, chap 1: 1-34.

6. Na GY, Suh MK, Sung YO et al. A decreased growth rate of the great toenail observed in patients with distal subungual onychomycosis. Ann Dermatol (Kor) 1995; 7: 217-221.

7. Goulden V, Goodfield MJD. Onychomycosis and linear nail growth. Br J Dermatol. 1997; 136: 139-140.

8. Baran R, Badillet G. Primary onycholysis of the big toenails, a review of 113 cases. Br J Dermatol. 1982; 106: 529-534.

9. Baran R, Dawber RPR, Tosti A, Haneke E. A text atlas of nail disorders. Martin Dunitz (London) 1996, chap 9, 169-193.

10. Zaias N, Drachman D. A method for the determination of drug effectiveness in onychomycosis. J Am Acad Dermatol. 1983; 9: 912-919.

11. Hay RJ, Clayton YM, Moore MK. Comparison of tioconazole 28% nail solution versus base as an adjunct to oral griseofulvin in patients with onychomycosis. Clin Exp Dermatol. 1987; 12: 175-177.

7.1 Topical treatment

Historically, topical nail therapy has met with little success, due in part to the absence of effective topical products. This is regrettable since there are potential candidates for topical therapy such as for fungal infections where potent systemic therapy is undesirable because of toxic effects or drug interactions. In addition, some patients may be unable or unwilling to take oral drugs for the many months of therapy required to ensure successful therapy, especially when only a few nails are affected. Therefore effective topical therapy directly applied to the nail plate would be an attractive alternative with the additional benefit of a complete absence of systemic side-effects and drug interactions. However, many of the conventional formulations of the antifungal agents (powders, solutions, creams, ointments) are not specifically adapted for use in the nails due to insufficient adhesion of the base, leading to insufficient penetration of the active ingredient through the nail into the nail bed; they are also not formulated to take account of the length of time which would be required to permit the growth of a healthy nail ; they also do not remain in contact with the site of application for long enough (they are readily removed by rubbing, wiping, washing).

Improvement of the conventional formulations led to the development of an alcoholic solution containing 28% tioconazole and undecylenic acid, for instance, which has produced moderate results [1]. Penetration of the drug, tioconazole, through the plate is excellent, but not matched by clinical efficacy.

7.1.1 Transungual drug delivery systems (TUDDS)

A further step forward has been achieved with the development of new vehicles in the form of colourless nail lacquers derived from cosmetic formulations. Two compounds, amorolfine and ciclopirox, are currently used in a lacquer base in several countries. These formulations fulfil two essential prerequisites : first, the active ingredient is in contact with the nail for long periods. Second, through evaporation of the solvents, the concentration of the active ingredient in the remaining film reservoir increases, thus providing the high concentration gradient essential for maximal penetration.

The amorolfine concentration in the film-forming solution is 5%; solvent evaporation leaves a film with a final amorolfine concentration of 19.8%. The ciclopirox concentration is 8% in the nail lacquer, increasing to 34.8% (Fig 7.1).

Fig 7.1
Schematic representation of transungual drug delivery system of ciclopirox nail lacquer

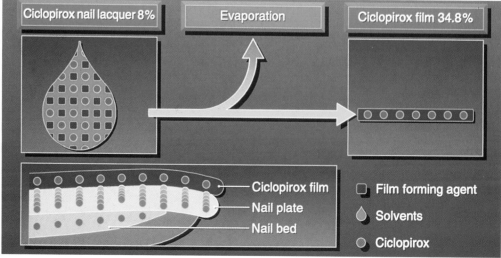

Fig 7.2
Ciclopirox.
Mode of action

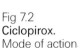

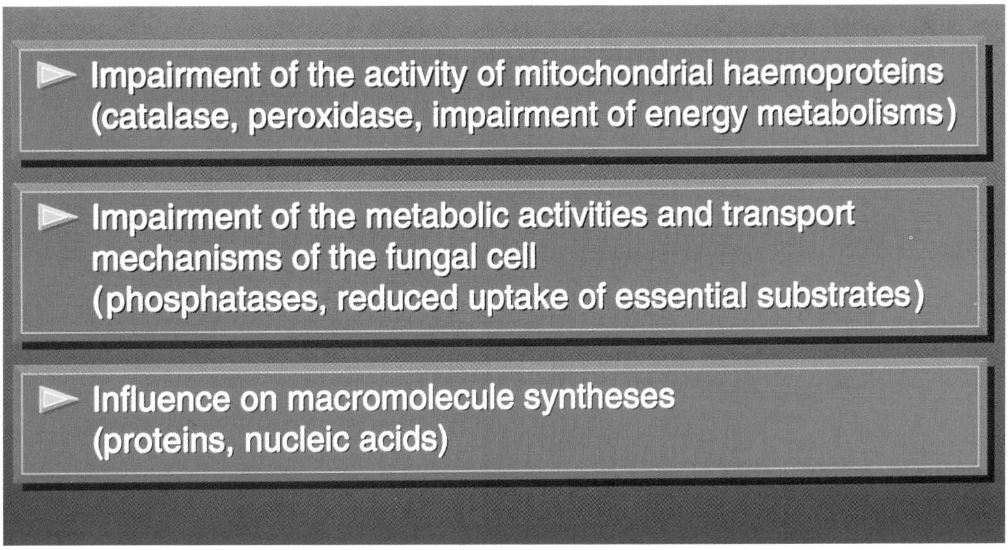

> **Impairment of the activity of mitochondrial haemoproteins (catalase, peroxidase, impairment of energy metabolisms)**

> **Impairment of the metabolic activities and transport mechanisms of the fungal cell (phosphatases, reduced uptake of essential substrates)**

> **Influence on macromolecule syntheses (proteins, nucleic acids)**

Release can be optimized by selecting the components of the lacquer formulation (solvent, polymer, plasticizer) which help to modulate the release of the drug and maintain the antifungal at a high level in the nail plate. Because of the additional occluding properties of these formulations, transungual water loss is reduced thus enhancing mass transport of the drug into and through the nail plate. Despite fulfilling all necessary prerequisites, diffusion may be disturbed in nails with fungal channels and splits, particularly at the border between the nail plate and the nail bed. This partially explains why cure is not always achieved.

Amorolfine belongs to a new family of anti-fungal drugs, the morpholines. Amorolfine inhibits two steps in the pathway of ergosterol biosynthesis namely the Δ14- reductase and the Δ7,8- isomerase which plays an important role in regulating membrane fluidity. This leads to accumulation of abnormal sterols and inhibits fungal growth. Amorolfine possesses a broad antimycotic spectrum against fungi pathogenic to plants and humans. In addition,

it shows strong fungicidal activity which is dependent on both concentration and time. Amorolfine is fungicidal against yeasts, dimorphic and dematiaceous fungi, but does not appear to be active against *Aspergillus, Fusarium* and *Mucor*.

Ciclopirox a hydroxy-pyridone derivative is incorporated in a clear nail lacquer containing poly (butyl hydrogen maleate, methoxyethylene) (1:1), ethylacetate, and 2-propanal [1a].

In contrast to most antifungals, it does not interfere with sterol biosynthesis (Fig 7.2). It acts as a chelating agent and primarily affects iron dependent mitochondrial enzymes(Fig 7.3). Consequently, as ciclopirox also impairs transport mechanisms into the fungal cell and in growing cells, there is reduced synthesis of macromolecules such as proteins and nucleic acids. Ciclopirox is characterized by a com-parably strong and broad fungicidal and sporicidal activity against the whole spectrum of human fungal pathogens at concentrations close to MIC.

Fig 7.3
Ciclopirox-iron (Fe^{3+}) complex

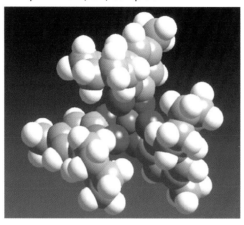

Its spectrum includes fungi such as *Scytalidium* and *Fusarium* spp. which are resistant to many other antifungals used in the treatment of onychomycosis. At therapeutically relevant concentrations, the spectrum of activity covers, in addition, gram-positive and gram-negative bacteria.

TUDDS is a new method of delivery which leads to penetration of mycotic nail keratin more rapidly than healthy nails. However the effectiveness of exclusively topical antimycotic treatment depends on the type of onychomycosis. PSO and TDO cannot be affected by topical treatment. This is considered to be the most appropriate therapy for SO. In the case of DLSO the cure rate depends largely upon the severity of nail infection. Where more than 60% of the nail plate is altered topical monotherapy is generally ineffective [2].

Clinical studies

In the framework of three large studies 714 patients with onychomycosis without matrix involvement applied amorolfine nail lacquer once weekly for 6 months (Fig 7.4,5). Mycological cure including negative culture and microscopy was achieved in 52.1% of the 424 toenail, and in 64.3% of the 98 fingernail mycoses. Local adverse events, mostly skin irritation, were reported in 6 patients (<1%) [3].

In an open multicentre study in 250 practices 5401 nails from 1239 patients were treated with the 8% ciclopirox lacquer formulation applied once daily to the affected nails over a treatment period of up to 6 months (Fig 7.6,7). The layer of lacquer was removed once weekly.

Fig 7.4
Onychomycosis sparing lunula
before treatment

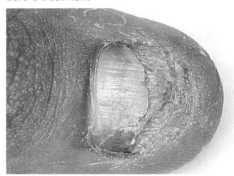

Fig 7.5
Onychomycosis sparing lunula
after treatment with amorolfine nail lacquer for 6 months

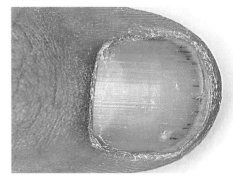

Fig 7.6
Onychomycosis of the great toenail
before treatment

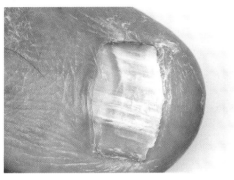

Fig 7.7
Onychomycosis of the great toenail
after treatment with ciclopirox nail lacquer

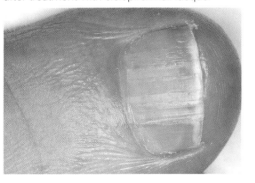

Fig 7.8
Lateral nail disease

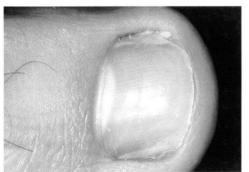

A cure was obtained in more than 50% of cases with a 60% success rate for fingernails. Only 2% of patients complained of periungual burning and redness [4]. In a recent study [5] it has been shown that under normal circumstances, one or two weekly applications of ciclopirox was as efficient as the former daily treatment.

In summary: topical treatment is suitable for SWO and early DLSO. The responses of patients with non extensive nail disease involving multiple nails are usually not as good. In addition, it is necessary to treat infected skin sites separately.

7.1.2 Nail avulsion

Filing and trimming of the nail performed by the patient are seldom helpful measures for treating subungual onychomycosis. On the other hand removal of as much diseased nail as possible by a dermatologist or podiatrist is helpful, but only as an adjunct to oral or topical antifungals [6]. It is a logical approach to eradicate the pathogen from lateral nail disease [7] (Fig 7.8-10) and from onycholytic pockets or canals (Fig 7.11) on the undersurface of the nail, which are sometimes filled with necrotic keratin and large compact amounts of fungi (dermatophytoma) [8, 9] (Fig 7.12). These factors are frequently responsible for the failure of systemic antifungals. Additionally impaired host immune response, inadequate absorption or distribution of the drug and inactivation, interaction or resistance to therapy may play a part. As in the case of dermatophyte nail infections, nail plate avulsion is also helpful in treating onychomycosis caused by yeasts and non-dermatophyte moulds [10–11].

It is mandatory to obtain a preoperative history and perform a clinical examination to eliminate contra-indications to local anaesthesia and/or nail surgery. Adequate anaesthesia, haemostasis and sterile techniques are prerequisites to surgery.

Total surgical nail avulsion [6,12]

Total nail avulsion can be carried out using either a distal or a proximal approach. In the usual technique for a distal approach (Fig 7.13) a Freer elevator or a dental spatula is used to detach the nail plate from the tissue to which it adheres i.e. the proximal nail fold and the nail bed. The operator proceeds by anterior-posterior movements (in order not to injure the longitudinal ridges of the nail bed). The detachment is completed by firmly pushing the instrument in the postero-lateral angles. Then, one of the lateral edges is grasped with a sturdy haemostat, in an upwards circular movement to accomplish removal of the nail. The proximal approach (Fig 7.14) for nail avulsion is advised when the subungual distal area adheres strongly to the nail plate and the hyponychium can be injured by introducing the spatula. The proximal nail fold is freed in the usual manner. Then the spatula is used to reflect the proximal nail fold, and is delicately inserted under the base of the nail plate where adherence is weak. The instrument is advanced distally following the natural cleavage plane, and this operation is repeated on the entire width of the subungual region. After freeing the last attachments, the nail plate is pulled out easily. Incidental to removing the nail plate, it is imperative that the nail bed and nail grooves be debrided of subungual debris; this is best accomplished by wiping the nail bed and nail grooves with a gauze wrapped around the end of a mosquito haemostat.

Fig 7.9
Lateral nail disease

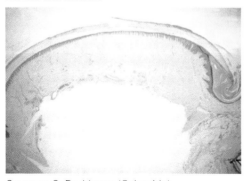

Courtesy G. Rodriguez (Colombia)

Fig 7.10
Lateral nail disease

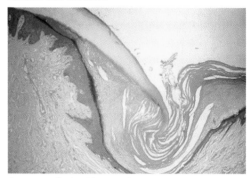

Courtesy G. Rodriguez (Colombia)
Acta Derm Venereol 1996; 73: 82-3
(with permission)

Fig 7.11
DLSO due to fungal leuconychia

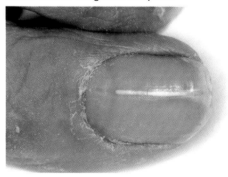

Fig 7.12
Dermatophytoma

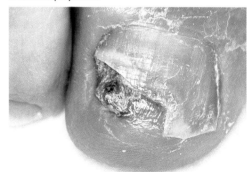

Total surgical removal has to be discouraged: the distal nail bed may shrink and become dislocated dorsally. In addition, the loss of counter-pressure produced by the removal of the nail plate allows expansion of the distal soft tissue and the distal edge of the regrowing nail then embeds itself (Fig 7.15). This can be largely overcome by using partial nail avulsion. However, in a small percentage of cases depending on the degree of patient discomfort, for example, when total surgical removal has been decided, the patient should be instructed to use a prosthetic nail on the regrowing nail plate so that the width of the nail bed is maintained and subsequent ingrowth is avoided [12].

Partial surgical nail avulsion [13]

Partial surgical nail avulsion for onychomycosis can be performed under local anaesthesia in a selected group of patients in whom the fungal infection is of limited extent. It permits the removal of the affected portion of the nail plate in one session, even when the disease has reached the buried region of the nail bed beneath the proximal nail fold.

The diseased nail plate including a margin of normal appearing nail is cut with an English nail splitter or a double action bone rongeur, then removed with sturdy forceps as for total avulsion. The digit is bandaged and postoperative care is continued for a few days [14].

In **DLSO**, surgery consists of removing the lateral or medial segment of the nail plate, especially on the toes (Fig 7.16a, b, c). Therefore enough normal nail is left to counteract the upward forces exerted on the distal soft tissue when walking and this will prevent the appearance of a distal nail wall.

Fig 7.13
Surgical nail removal.
Distal avulsion

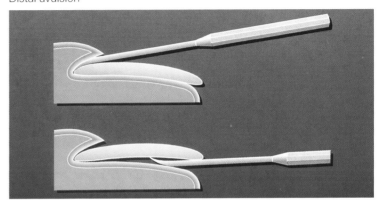

Fig 7.14
Surgical nail removal.
Proximal avulsion

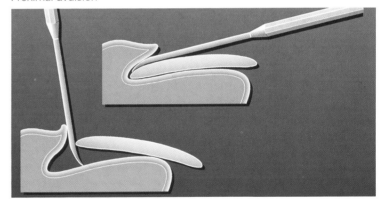

Fig 7.15
Risk of total nail avulsion.
Normal toe   Toe after nail plate avulsion

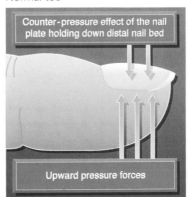

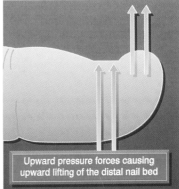

Fig 7.16a
Surgery of distal lateral subungual
onychomycosis

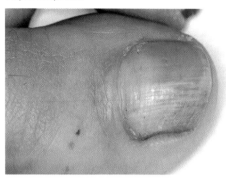

In *Candida* **onycholysis,** thorough clipping
away of as much of the detached nail as
possible facilitates the daily application of an
antifungal drug until nail growth is achieved
(Fig 7.17).

In **proximal subungual onychomycosis**
removal of the non-adherent base of the nail
plate is easy (Fig 7.18, 19). The nail plate is
detached from the proximal nail fold. The lunula
region of the nail is then cut transversally with a
nail splitter by inserting the instrument beneath
the lateral edge of the nail. Leaving the distal
portion of the nail in place decreases discomfort. As for DLSO, in any type of onychomycosis treated surgically, the avulsed
segment must always include a margin of
normal nail.

Fig 7.16b
Surgery of distal lateral subungual
onychomycosis

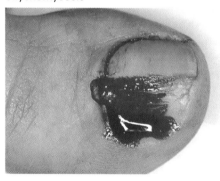

Recalcitrant *Candida* paronychia with
secondary nail plate invasion may be treated by
surgical excision of a crescent of thickened
proximal nail fold associated with partial
avulsion of the affected portion of the nail
keratin [15] (Fig 7.20-22).

Chemical avulsion

Chemical avulsion is a painless method
which has superseded partial surgical avulsion.
It may be repeated as often as necessary.
The formulation used is shown in Table 7.1
[16].

Fig 7.16c
Surgery of distal lateral subungual
onychomycosis

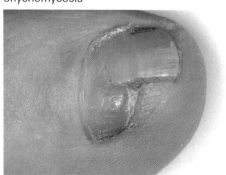

Table 7.1
Urea ointment formulation

Urea	40 percent
White beeswax (or paraffin)	5 percent
Anhydrous lanolin	20 percent
White petrolatum	25 percent
Silica gel type H	10 percent

Fig 7.17
Candida onycholysis

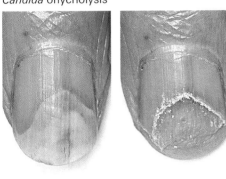

Fig 7.18
Partial surgical nail avulsion in proximal subungual onychomycosis

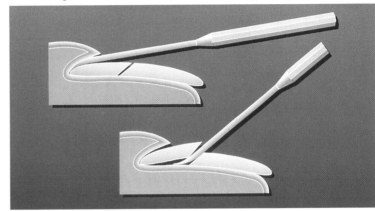

Fig 7.19
Surgical nail removal

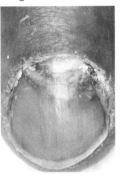
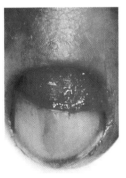

Fig 7.21
Treatment of recalcitrant chronic paronychia

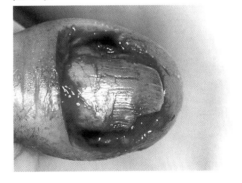

Fig 7.20
Treatment of recalcitrant chronic paronychia

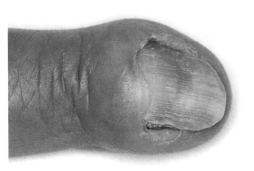

Fig 7.22
Treatment of recalcitrant chronic paronychia

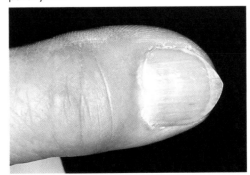

Urea ointment is applied to the nail plate after protecting the surrounding skin e.g. with adhesive dressing. The entire distal digit is then wrapped for a week (Fig 7.23-25).

Urea ointment appears to act on the bond between the nail keratin and the diseased nail bed; it spares only the normal nail tissue. Afterwards, blunt dissection using a nail elevator and nail clipper leaves the remaining portion of normal nail plate intact. Following removal of the diseased part of the nail, topical antifungal agents (imidazoles, tolnaftate, haloprogin, ciclopiroxolamine) should be applied for several months under occlusion, especially if there is no associated systemic therapy. Combination 20% urea and 10% salicylic acid ointment has been suggested [17].

Some authors prefer using 50% potassium iodide ointment in anhydrous lanolin plus 0.5% iodochlorhydroxyquine instead of 40% urea for keratinolysis [18].

A ready-made topical preparation containing 40% urea and 1% bifonazole is available [19, 20]. This preparation is applied under occlusion and the patient is asked to debride the nails every day for 1–2 weeks, facilitating removal of the diseased nail keratin within 1 or 2 weeks of this daily treatment. Then, 1% bifonazole cream is applied once a day for 2 months to the whole nail area and rubbed onto the nail bed. In some clinical trials, the efficacy of this ointment has been demonstrated provided that the instructions are properly followed and that strict compliance by the patient is ensured [19, 20]. However, such treatment is difficult to apply in the elderly, tedious when several digits are affected and/or ineffective when the proximal portion of the nail plate is invaded by fungal organisms beneath the nail fold. Once again, the treatment is more suitable for limited and early nail disease. The unpleasant odour following use of urea ointment, especially when left for 1 week, has lead to the development of a new formulation still under investigation, which may resolve most of the problems due to the chemical keratinolysis.

Fig 7.23
Chemical avulsion with urea/bifonazole

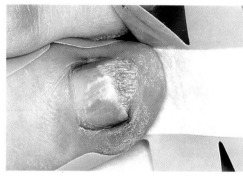

Fig 7.24

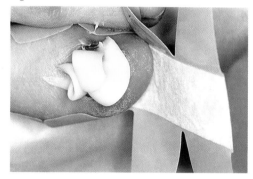

Fig 7.25

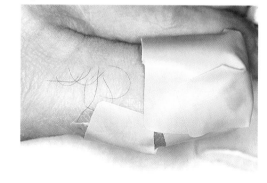

References

1. Hay RJ, Mackie RM, Clayton YM. Tioconazole nail solution – an open study of its efficacy in onychomycosis. Clin Exp Dermatol. 1985; 10: 111–115.

1a. Ciclopirox nail lacquer: the first prescription topical therapy for onychomycosis. J Am Acad Dermatol 2000; 43 (Suppl 4): S55–56; S57–69; S70–80; S81–95; S96–102.

2. Effendy I. Therapeutic strategies in onychomycosis. JEADV 1995; 4 (Suppl 1): S3–S10.

3. Zaug M. Amorolfine nail lacquer: clinical experience in onychomycosis. JEADV 1995; 4 (Suppl 1): S23–S30

4. Seebacher C, Ulbricht H, Wörz K. Results of a multicentre study with ciclopirox nail lacquer in patients with onychomycosis. Hautnah Myk. 1993; 3: 80–84.

5. Nolting S, Ulbricht H. Untersuchungen zur Applikationsfrequenz von Ciclopirox-lack (8%) bei der Behandlung von Onychomycosen. Jatros Derma 1997; 11: 20–26.

6. Baden HP. Treatment of distal onychomycosis with avulsion and topical antifungal agents under occlusion. Arch Dermatol. 1994; 130: 558–559.

7. Baran R, de Donker P. Lateral edge nail involvement indicates poor prognosis for treating onychomycosis with the new systemic antifungals. Acta Derm Venereol. 1996; 76: 82–83.

8. Hay RJ. Chronic dermatophyte infections. In: Superficial fungal infections. Verbov J.(ed). MTP Press Limited, Lancaster (England) 1986, p 23–24.

9. Roberts DT, Evans EGV. Subungual dermatophytoma complicating dermatophyte onychomycosis. Br J Dermatol. 1998; 138: 189–190.

10. Baran R, Tosti A, Piraccini BM. Uncommon clinical patterns of Fusarium nail infection: report of three cases. Br J Dermatol. 1997; 136: 424–427.

11. Rollman O, Johansson S. *Hendersonula toruloidea* infection: Successful response of onychomycosis to nail avulsion and topical ciclopiroxolamine. Acta Dermato Venereol. 1987; 67: 506–510.

12. Dominguez-Cherit J, Teixeira F, Arenas R. Combined surgical and systemic treatment of onychomycosis. Br J Dermatol. 1999 (in press).

13. Baran R, Hay RJ. Partial surgical avulsion of the nail in onychomycosis. Clin Exp Derm. 1985; 10:413–418.

14. Elewski BE, Hay RJ. Update on the management of onychomycosis: Highlights of the third annual summit on cutaneous antifungal therapy. Clin Infect Dis 1996; 23: 305–313.

15. Baran R, Bureau H. Surgical treatment of recalcitrant chronic paronychia of the fingers. J Dermatol Surg Oncol. 1981; 7: 106–107.

16. South DA, Farber EM. Urea ointment in non surgical avulsion of nail dystrophies. Reappraisal. Cutis 1980; 26: 609–612.

17. Buselmeier T. Combination urea and salicylic acid ointment nail avulsion in non dystrophic nails: Follow-up observation. Cutis 1980; 25: 397–405.

18. Dorn M, Kienitz T, Ryckmanns F. Onychomycosis: Experience with non traumatic nail avulsion. Hautarzt 1980; 31: 30–34.

19. Torres-Rodriguez JM, Madreny N, Nicolas MC. Non-traumatic topical treatment of onychomycosis with urea associated with bifonazole. Mycoses 1991; 34: 499–504.

20. Bonifaz A, Guzman A, Garcia C et al. Efficacy and safety of bifonazole urea in the two-phase treatment of onychomycosis. Int J Dermatol. 1995; 34: 500–503

Review of current antifungal therapy

7.2 Systemic treatment with new antifungal drugs

The efficacy of the new systemically active antifungal drugs – itraconazole, fluconazole and terbinafine – is clear (Table 7.2) but the frequency and seriousness of side effects should be an integral part of the decision on the use of a rational treatment [1].

We have therefore extensively reviewed the issue of safety, drug interactions, and the spectrum of adverse events.

Itraconazole

Pharmacology. Itraconazole is a triazole antifungal agent effective against dermatophytes, yeasts and many pathogenic moulds. It is a strong inhibitor of fungal ergosterol biosynthesis which is crucial for the correct functioning of fungal lipid membranes. It has a high affinity to fungal cytochrome P450 and only weakly binds to mammalian cytochrome P450-linked enzymes. Itraconazole has the broadest in vitro action spectrum of all available systemically active antifungal drugs [2]. In vitro resistance to itraconazole is rare.

Pharmacokinetics (Fig 7.26, 27). Itraconazole is a highly lipophilic substance and well absorbed from the gastrointestinal tract under acid conditions. It should be given directly after a meal. It is significantly better absorbed when administered in a cyclodextrin formulation, used for treatment of oropharyngeal candidosis in severely ill patients. Itraconazole is metabolized in the liver to inactive metabolites, 40% of which are excreted with the urine, the rest with faeces [5].

Itraconazole reaches the skin via passive diffusion from the dermal capillaries, massive excretion with sebum, and incorporation into basal keratinocytes, but little is found in sweat. Epidermis and nail concentrations are much higher than plasma levels. Itraconazole shows very strong binding to keratin. Redistribution of itraconazole from stratum corneum and nail into plasma is negligible. Nails take up and concentrate itraconazole. It can be detected in nail clippings as early as 7 days after the start of treatment. Within 1 month, higher concentrations are reached in finger than in toenails. Doubling the dose from 100 mg to 200 mg daily increased itraconazole nail concentrations seven to ten fold. High nail levels are maintained for 6 to 9 months in finger and toenails. Itraconazole nail concentrations appear to parallel cure rates. The drug is also found to be concentrated at the major site of infection, that is in the hyperkeratosis of the nail bed. Nail clippings had 240 ng/g whereas subungual hyperkeratosis showed concentrations of 567 ng/g [5,6].

Rapid appearance, concentration, and persistence of itraconazole in the nail plate were the rationale for the development of intermittent treatment with daily pulses of itraconazole 200 mg twice daily for one week per month for two to three times [7].

Adverse effects. Itraconazole is generally well tolerated. Adverse effects mainly involve gastrointestinal symptoms and skin alterations. Nausea, vomiting, abdominal pain, and diarrhoea occur in about 10%. Asymptomatic increase of liver enzymes is observed in 1 to 2%, but serious liver disease is rare. Ventricular fibrillation has been described due to itraconazole-induced hypokalaemia. Headaches were observed in 2.3%, and dizziness in 1.4%. A single case of thrombocytopenia and leukopenia has been described.

A case of acute generalized pustulosis has also been described, but the most frequent skin abnormalities are rashes with a frequency below 3%. Oedema is rare and may be due to interaction with nifedipine [2].

Drug interactions. Although less than ketoconazole, itraconazole has been shown to interact with a number of drugs. Some drugs decrease itraconazole levels dramatically by reducing its absorption from the GI tract (antacids, H_2 receptor blockers) or increasing and accelerating itraconazole biodegradation

Table 7.2
In vitro minimal inhibitory concentrations [µg/ml] for dermatophytes *cultured from onychomycoses* (first line: *T. rubrum, T. mentagrophytes, T. tonsurans, T. violaceum, T. soudanense, M. canis, E. floccosum* [3]; second line: *T. rubrum, T. mentagrophytes* [4])

Itraconazole	Fluconazole	Terbinafine
0.06 – 0.5	1 – 64	0.003 – 0.06
0.1 – 2	64 – 1024	0.001 – 0.05

Fig 7.26
Penetration pathways in the nail of the new oral antifungal drugs

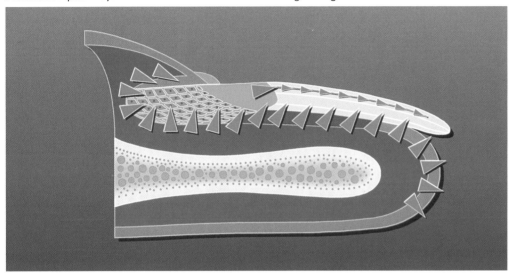

Fig 7.27
Itraconazole content in the distal nail plate (100 mg o.d. for 3 months)

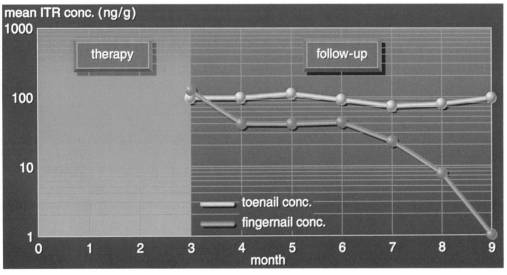

(particularly rifampicin, phenytoin, and others). Itraconazole increases drug levels or activity of H_1-antagonists such as terfenadine and astemizole, phenytoin, oral antidiabetic substances, oral anticoagulants, hypnotic agents, methyl-prednisolone, cyclosporin, digoxin, hypolipidaemic substances, etc [8]. Acute rhabdomyolysis has been induced by a lovastatin-itraconazole interaction. Uveitis was caused by itraconazole-induced high levels of rifabutin. Amaurosis and vomiting occurred under digoxin treatment. It may enhance toxicity of anticancer drugs, but it was also shown to reverse multidrug resistance in acute leukaemias. The levels of antipyrine and possibly oral contraceptives may be lowered by itraconazole (Table 7.3).

Review of current antifungal therapy

Table 7.3
Drug interactions with the new antifungal drugs [8,9]

Itraconazole	Fluconazole	Terbinafine
Drugs increasing levels of antimycotic		
	Hydrochlorothiazide Other thiazide diuretics?	Cimetidine
Drugs decreasing levels of antimycotic		
Rifampicin Isoniazid Phenytoin Phenobarbitone Carbamazepine H_2-antagonists Antacids Didanosine (due to its high pH buffer in the tablet formulation) Anticholinergic drugs	Rifampicin	Rifampicin Phenobarbital
Drugs whose activity or levels may be increased		

Phenytoin
Warfarin
H_1-antagonists
   Terfenadine
   Astemizole
Digoxin
Alprazolam
Triazolam
Midazolam
Felodipine
Fluoxetine
Nifedipine
Corticosteroids
   Methylprednisolone
Cyclosporin A
Cisapride
Zidovudine
Protease inhibitors
Busulfan
Vincristine
Oral antidiabetic drugs (sulphonyl urea)
   Tolbutamide
   Glibenclamide
   Glipizide
Lovastatin
Simvastatin
Quinidine
	Warfarin*
	Phenytoin*
	H_1-antagonists?*
	   Astemizole
	   Terfenadine
	Midazolam*
	Triazolam*
	Nortriptyline
	Theophylline
	Rifabutin*
	Zidovudine
	Cyclosporin A*
		Warfarin
		Nortriptyline
		Nicotinamide

Drugs that may be decreased in activity/safety		
Oral contraceptives?	Oral contraceptives? Antipyrine	

* Drug interactions are usually less severe with fluconazole than with itraconazole

Precautions. Due to its interaction with many other drugs metabolized by cytochrome P450-linked enzymes, itraconazole should be used cautiously in elderly patients who are often on multidrug therapy.

Itraconazole rarely causes hepatic reactions. A baseline liver function test is only recommended in patients with a history of liver disease, potentially hepatotoxic drugs and excessive alcohol consumption.

Itraconazole dosing. Itraconazole is given either as a 200 mg dose once daily [10] for 3 months or, preferably, as a pulse therapy with intermittent dosing of 200 mg itraconazole twice daily for 1 week each month over a period of 2 months for fingernail and three months for toenail fungal infections.

Itraconazole in onychomycosis
(Fig 7.28, 29). Since itraconazole is rapidly distributed to the nails, then accumulated, concentrated and retained in the nails for many months, intermittent treatment using a dose of 200 mg twice daily over 1 week per month was instituted giving the same good results while reducing the amount of drug given as well as the drug cost by 50% [11]. Intermittent treatment is well tolerated, safe, as effective as continuous therapy with 200 mg daily, and less expensive [12]. Relapse rates are approximately 10% [13]. A combination of itraconazole with ciclopirox nail lacquer in very severe cases clearly surpasses the results of systemic monotherapy [14].

Fluconazole

Pharmacology. Fluconazole is a bis-triazole antifungal agent effective against systemic and superficial mycoses. It is an inhibitor of fungal lanosterol 14a-demethylase which is a cytochrome P450-dependent enzyme [15]. Fluconazole has particularly been used to treat yeast infections but is also very active against dermatophyte infections [16] (Table 7.2). However, its in vitro activity is relatively low and in vitro tests do not reliably predict the clinical value of fluconazole for dermatophyte infections. It can inhibit germ tube formation of *C. albicans* spores in remarkably low concentrations [Haneke, unpublished]. Its efficacy depends on the daily dose, on corresponding plasma and tissue levels, the susceptibility of

Fig 7.28
Onychomycosis before treatment

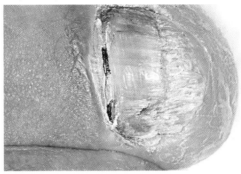

Fig 7.29
Onychomycosis after treatment
with itraconazole

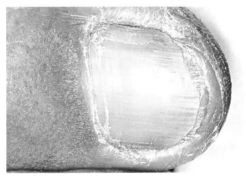

the fungi and, above all, on the immune competence of the patient.

Resistance to fluconazole has been observed [17], mainly in AIDS patients with candidosis [18]. The mechanism may be reduced azole uptake which appears to be fluconazole-specific, or through an increased fungal cytochrome P450 level which counteracts the effect of all azole antifungals. Other mechanisms include increased efflux of drug from the cell or altered cell membrane biosynthesis.

Pharmacokinetics [19, 20]. Fluconazole is a hydrophilic and relatively keratinophilic substance (Table 7.4). Its bioavailability is over 90% and it is neither dependent on gastric pH nor the presence of food, antacids, or histamine H$_2$-receptor antagonists. It reaches the stratum corneum and the nails by diffusion from dermal vessels. It is excreted with sweat, but is virtually absent from sebum. It is retained and concentrated in stratum corneum [21] and nails [22]. It is 2 to 3 times more slowly eliminated from stratum corneum than from plasma. Higher levels are reached in healthy nails than in fungus infected nails and these remain detectable for 3 to 6 months after the end of treatment [22]. The concentrations reached are well above the MICs of most dermatophytes.

Fluconazole undergoes extensive tubular reabsorption and consequently has a long elimination half-life permitting once daily dosing.

In children fluconazole appears to have a shorter plasma half-life and a larger volume of distribution than in adult patients [18].

Table 7.4
Pharmacology and pharmacokinetic properties of itraconazole, fluconazole and terbinafine

	Itraconazole	Fluconazole	Terbinafine
Chemistry	triazole	bis-triazole	allylamine
	lipophilic, highly keratinophilic	hydrophilic, keratinophilic	lipophilic, strongly keratinophilic
Pharmacology			
Action mechanism	inhibition of ergosterol synthesis (lanosterol-demethylase)	inhibition of ergosterol synthesis (lanosterol-demethylase)	inhibition of ergosterol synthesis (squalene-epoxidase)
Cytochrome P450 dependent	yes	yes	no
Effect of human sterol biosynthesis	weak	almost none	none
Resistance development	very rare	rare	not reported
Pharmacokinetics			
Absorption	requires acid pH	independent of pH and food intake	independent of food intake
Peak plasma concentrations	289 ng/ml, 4.7 h after 200 mg	reached after 3 hours	after 2 hours
Plasma protein binding	>99%	12%	>98%
Metabolism in liver	extensive	virtually none	extensive
Excretion	40% urine, rest with faeces	completely with urine	80% with urine
Diffusion to skin	capillary vessels, excretion with sebum, incorporation in basal cells	capillaries, excretion with sweat, incorporation in basal cells	capillaries, excretion with sebum, weakly with sweat, incorporation in basal cells
Drug in nails	concentration and persistence for 6 to 9 months, concentration in subungual keratoses	rapid appearance, concentration, persistence for 3 to 6 months	rapid appearance, concentration, persistence for 3 to 6 months

Adverse effects. In dosages up to 400 mg/ day given for at least 7 days, the incidence of adverse effects was 16%. However, at least one third of these patients had AIDS, and it is not clear what was due to the disease, concomitant medication, or fluconazole. Half of the side effects are gastrointestinal complaints: nausea 3.7%, abdominal pain 1.7%, vomiting 1.7%, diarrhoea 1.5%. Headache and skin rash were the other most frequent untoward effects with 1.9% and 1.8%, respectively. Discontinuation of treatment was necessary in 1.5%. Asymptomatic elevations of liver enzymes are estimated to occur in less than 5%. One patient with pre-existing hepatic disease developed hepatitis that resolved after withdrawal of fluconazole. Other isolated events have been fatal acute hepatic necrosis, agranulocytosis, seizures, adrenal insufficiency, thrombocytopenia. High doses of fluconazole during pregnancy have been related to congenital anomalies.

Serious dermatological adverse effects include Lyell's syndrome and Stevens-Johnson syndrome including one death in an AIDS patient; the true cause is, however, obscured by the serious illness and the concomitant multidrug therapy. A fixed drug eruption considered to be a localized form of toxic epidermal necrolysis, has been described once. Drug rashes appear to be particularly frequent in AIDS patients. Eleven of 26 Mycosis Study Group Centres in the USA reported a total of 33 patients with severe, reversible alopecia; 29 of 33 patients (88%) received at least 400 mg of fluconazole daily for an average of 1 month.

Drug interactions. Fluconazole inhibits fungal cytochrome P450 associated enzymes, but mammalian cytochrome P450 is also affected in doses >200 mg/day. Fluconazole plasma levels are considerably decreased when rifampicin is given concomitantly. Fluconazole increases drug levels and intensifies the action of many other drugs [18]. Theophylline clearance may be decreased (Table 7.3).

Fluconazole dosing. Fluconazole is given in a dose of 50 to 100 mg/day for skin mycoses. For onychomycoses, a once-weekly dose of 300 mg is recommended. Treatment duration is 6 months for toenails and three months for fingernails.

Fluconazole in onychomycosis. Fluconazole has been shown to be retained and concentrated in keratinous structures [23] which is the rationale for intermittent dosing. It is given once a week. Because of its rapid penetration into the nail a one-day administration per week is sufficient. It was shown that fluconazole was present in cured nails in high concentrations 3 and 6 months after the end of treatment and the concentrations were higher than those of itraconazole and terbinafine [23].

Several studies have shown promising results using 150 mg orally once weekly over 6 to 12 months [24-27], but for better results 300 mg once weekly for 6 months is required [25]. A traditional regimen of 100 mg/day for 6 months gave however a success rate of 80%, and a similar dose given every other day was also successful, even in patients who either did not respond to, or did not tolerate griseofulvin [27]. Fluconazole has also been combined with nail removal using urea.

Terbinafine

Pharmacology. Terbinafine is the first orally active allylamine antifungal. It is a specific inhibitor of fungal squalene epoxidase which blocks ergosterol synthesis that is necessary for the integrity of the fungal cell membrane [28]. Its activity against *Candida* appears to be species-dependent with fungicidal action against *C. parapsilosis,* but it is fungistatic against *C. albicans.* It is also active against some non-dermatophyte moulds [29].

Pharmacokinetics. Terbinafine is well absorbed from the gastrointestinal tract. Its bioavailability is usually over 70% [29]. Terbinafine is highly lipophilic, strongly binds to plasma proteins in a non-specific manner, and is keratinophilic (Table 7.4). It is accumulated in the adipose tissue giving a depot effect and slow elimination from the body. The nail is reached by diffusion from the dermal vessels and incorporation into basal keratinocytes. Terbinafine appears in the horny layer within 24 hours after the first dose attaining therapeutically active concentrations in skin, nails, hair and sebum. Terbinafine reaches the nail via nail bed and matrix by diffusion and via the matrix by incorporation into the growing onychocytes [30]. After 7 days, drug concentrations were 0.43 µg/g in peripheral nail clippings exceeding minimal inhibitory concentrations of most dermatophytes 10 to 100 times [31].

Terbinafine is slowly eliminated from nails after discontinuation of treatment. Almost half of the drug concentration is still retained for 90 days at levels higher than the MIC values of most nail pathogens by a factor of 5 to 50 times. The long-term accumulation of terbinafine enables a relatively short period of treatment for eradication of fungal nail infections.

Terbinafine biotransformation is reduced in hepatic disease and the terminal half-life increases in renal insufficiency [29].

Adverse effects. Adverse effects are rare and mostly slight and transient. Gastrointestinal (incidence 5.2%), cutaneous (2.7%), and central nervous system side effects (1.2%) prevail. A postmarketing study of 9879 patients revealed that 14.5% of patients reported some medical events, 49% of which were thought to be possibly or probably related to terbinafine. Less than 1% were serious and only 5 of these were related to treatment [32]. Gastrointestinal symptoms include irritation, dyspepsia, nausea, vomiting, diarrhoea, cramps, gastric fullness, and nausea. Taste alterations, typically occurring 5 to 8 weeks after starting oral terbinafine are experienced by 0.12 to 0.6% of patients, mainly as hypogeusia, ageusia, cacogeusia and metallic taste. The taste disturbance usually resolves within 4 months after withdrawal. Smell disturbance, discoloration [33] and burning of the tongue appear to be rare. Headache, dizziness, lack of concentration, sleeplessness, and other central nervous system effects occur in about 1.2%. Green vision was recently observed.

Skin side effects include rashes, urticaria, serum sickness–like reaction, pruritus, eczema, erthroderma, and development or exacerbation of psoriasis (Table 7.5).

Serious side effects are rare, but may be life-threatening. Decreased numbers of blood cells and agranulocytosis are rare as is terbinafine-induced hepatic disease [34]. Renal impairment due to terbinafine appears to be exceptional. Severe adverse effects affecting the skin include acute generalized exanthematous pustulosis, severe erythema multiforme, Stevens-Johnson syndrome [35], and toxic epidermal necrolysis [36]. In patients with onychomycosis, the German medical profession drug advisory board therefore recommends first considering a topical treatment and prescribing oral terbinafine treatment only after a very careful risk-benefit consideration [37]. Other authorities do not take this view.

Drug interactions. Interactions with other drugs are remarkably rare, probably because terbinafine does not have a high affinity for liver microsome cytochrome P450 enzymes (Table 7.3). Cimetidine may increase terbinafine levels and rifampicin and phenobarbitone were found to decrease them. Terbinafine decreases cyclosporin A levels in blood possibly by inducing a metabolic degradation of cyclo-sporin A; however, this does not require a dose adjustment.

Precautions. Although routine laboratory monitoring is probably not necessary in patients without a history of liver disease and haematological disorders it is wise to have a baseline liver function test and blood count in patients at risk, especially when there is a history of hepatitis, heavy drinking, blood dyscrasias, etc.

Terbinafine dosing. Terbinafine is given in a dose of 250 mg per day in adults. A treatment duration of 6 weeks is deemed sufficient for fingernail and of 12 weeks for toenail fungal infections.

Terbinafine in onychomycosis (Fig 7.30,31). Initially terbinafine was given as long as the affected nails took to regrow healthy. Because of the good results and its persistence in the nail for 3 months after the end of therapy the treatment period was shortened. Cure rates were 71% and 79% after 12 and 24 weeks of treatment, respectively [38]. Early studies suggested clearance rates of 95% for fingernail and 82% for toenail onychomycosis. Prolongation of terbinafine treatment duration from 3 to 6 months did not improve the mycological cure rate and clinical cure rates [39]. A follow-up examination of 22 patients of this study 2 ½ years later revealed that nearly half of the patients had a clinical and mycological cure.

A double-blind comparison with griseofulvin showed 79% complete cures with 3 months' terbinafine compared to 39% for griseofulvin after 3 months of treatment for fingernail mycoses [40]. A 24-week course of terbinafine was also significantly more effective than a 48-week course of griseofulvin in toenail dermatophytosis.

The first study comparing itraconazole 200 mg daily with terbinafine 250 mg daily, did not show significantly different cure rates [41]. However the follow-up period of this study was only 6 months. Another comparative study of

250 mg terbinafine daily for 12 weeks versus itraconazole 200 mg daily for 12 weeks showed terbinafine to be superior after a follow-up period of 40 weeks [42]. In toenail onychomycosis caused by dermatophytes, a double-blind comparative trial of terbinafine 250 mg/day versus itraconazole 200 mg/day (186 patients in each group) showed at week 48 that terbinafine produced higher rates of clinical and mycological cure than did itraconazole [43]. Two studies have shown that terbinafine given as weekly pulses of 500 mg daily once a month is as effective as continuous treatment with 250 mg daily and itraconazole pulse therapy [44].

A more recent multicentre European study compared continuous terbinafine at 250 mg daily for 3 or 4 months against pulsed itraconazole at 400 mg daily for 1 week repeated monthly for 3 or 4 months. At follow-up 56 weeks later there were significantly more patients in mycological remission amongst those taking terbinafine for both 3 and 4 months compared to those on the 3 or 4 pulse regimen of itraconazole [45].

Although its in vitro activity against *Scopulariopsis brevicaulis* is high, its clinical efficacy is unpredictable. *Candida parapsilosis* nail infections were effectively treated whereas *C. albicans* required 500 mg per day and a longer duration of treatment. Combined treatment using atraumatic removal of the diseased nail plate allows clinicians to use shorter courses of therapy. We have shown that a combination of terbinafine with topical application of amorolfine nail lacquer increased the overall cure rate [46].

Pharmaco-economic aspects of oral onychomycosis treatment. The cost of treatment of onychomycoses is far more than just the cost of the drug. Treatment duration, physician consultations, administrative cost, mycology and laboratory examinations are all factors, and cure, as well as relapse rates are further important aspects. Depending on the method used to calculate cost-benefit, both terbinafine and itraconazole have been suggested to be the most cost-effective systemic drugs [47].

Fig 7.30
Onychomycosis due to *T. rubrum* before treatment

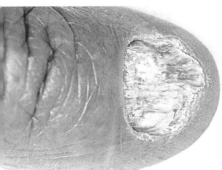

Fig 7.31
Onychomycosis at 6 months, following 1 month's treatment with terbinafine

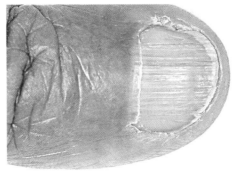

References

1. Haneke E. The potential risks of not treating onychomycosis. In: Proceedings of the 2nd International Symposium on Onychomycosis, Florence 1995. Macclesfield, Cheshire: Gardiner-Caldwell Comm Ltd 1966: 12–14
2. Grant SM, Clissold SP. Itraconazole. A review of its pharmacodynamic and pharmacokinetic properties, and therapeutic use in superficial and systemic mycoses. Drugs 1989; 37:310–344

3. Clayton YM. *In vitro* activity of terbinafine. Clin Exp Dermatol 1989; 14:101–103
4. Korting HC, Ollert M, Abeck D, German Collab Dermatophyte Drug Susceptibility Group. Results of a German multicenter study on drug susceptibility of *Trichophyton rubrum* and *Trichophyton mentagrophytes* isolated from tinea unguium. Antimicrob Agents Chemother 1995; 39:1206–1208
5. Haria M, Bryson HM, Goa KL. Itraconazole. A reappraisal of its pharmacological properties and thera-

peutic use in the management of superficial fungal infections. Drugs 1996; 51:585–620
6. De Doncker P. Pharmacokinetics in onychomycosis. In Jacobs PH, Nall L, eds. Fungal Disease. Biology, Immunology, and Diagnosis. New York: M Dekker; 1997:517–543
7. De Doncker P, Decroix J, Piérard GE, Roelant D, Woestenborghs R, Jacqmin P, Odds F, Heremans A, Dockx P, Roseeuw D. Antifungal pulse therapy in onychomycosis: a pharmacokinetic and pharmacodynamic investigation of monthly cycles of 1-week pulse with

itraconazole. Arch Dermatol 1996; 132:34–41

8. Roberts DT. The risk/benefit ratio of modern antifungal pharmacological agents. In: Aly R, Beutner KR, Maibach H. Cutaneous Infection and Therapy. New York: M Dekker, 1997:183–190

9. Brodell RT, Elewski BE. Clinical pearl: antifungal drugs and drug interactions. J Am Acad Dermatol 1995; 33: 259–260

10. Haneke E, Delescluse J, Plinck EPB, Hay RJ. The use of itraconazole in onychomycosis. Eur J Dermatol 1996; 6:7–10

11. Odom RB, Aly R, Scher RK, Daniel CR III, Elewski BE, Zaias N, DeVillez R, Jacko M, Oleka N, Moskovitz BL. A multicenter, placebo-controlled, double-blind study of intermittent therapy with itraconazole for the treatment of onychomycosis of the fingernail. J Am Acad Dermatol 1997; 36: 231–235

12. van Doorslaer EK, Tormans G, Gupta AK, van Rossem K, Eggleston A, Dubois DJ, de Doncker P, Haneke E. Economic evaluation of antifungal agents in the treatment of toenail onychomycosis in Germany. Dermatology 1996; 193:239–244

13. Hull PR. Onychomycosis – treatment, relapse and re-infection. Dermatology 1997; 194: Suppl 1:7–9

14. Nolting S.Satellite Symposium. Onychomycosis. New approaches in therapy. Proceedings 19th World Congress of Dermatology June 18, 1997, Sydney, Australia (in press).

15. Back DJ, Tjia JF, Abel SM. Azoles, allylamines and drug metabolism. Br J Dermatol 1992; 126: Suppl 39:14–18

16. Fischbein A, Haneke E, Lacner K, Male O, Mohn R, Muller H, O'Conolly M, Tronnier H. Comparative evaluation of oral fluconazole and oral ketoconazole in the treatment of fungal infections of the skin. Int J Dermatol 1992; 31: Suppl 2:12–16

17. Rex JH, Rinaldi MG, Pfaller MA. Resistance of Candida species to fluconazole. Antimicrob Agents Chemother 1995; 39:1–8

18. Goa KL, Barradell LB. Fluconazole. An update of its pharmacodynamic and pharmacokinetic properties and therapeutic use in major superficial and systemic mycoses in immunocompromised patients. Drugs 1995; 50:658–690

19. Rich P, Scher RK, Breneman D et al. Pharmacokinetics of three doses of once-weekly fluconazole (150, 300, and 450 mg) in distal subungual onychomycosis of the toenail. J Am Acad Dermatol. 1998; 38: S 103–109.

20. Savin RC, Drake L, Babel D et al. Pharmacokinetics of three once-weekly dosages of fluconazole (150, 300, or 450 mg) in distal subungual onychomycosis of the fingernail. J Am Acad Dermatol. 1998; 38: S 110–116.

21. Debruyne D. Clinical pharmacokinetics of fluconazole in superficial and systemic mycoses. Clin Pharmacokinet 1997; 33:52–77

22. Haneke E. Fluconazole levels in human epidermis and blister fluid. Br J Dermatol 1990; 123:273–274

23. Faergemann J, Laufen H. Levels of fluconazole in normal and diseased nails during and after treatment of onychomycoses in toe-nails with fluconazole 150 mg once weekly. Acta Derm Venereol 1996; 76:219–221

24. Gupta AK, Scher RK, Rich P. Fluconazole for the treatment of onychomycosis: an update. Int J Dermatol 1998; 37: 815–820.

25. Drake L, Babel D, Stewart D et al. Once-weekly fluconazole (150, 300 or 450 mg) in the treatment of distal subungual onychomycosis of the fingernail. J Am Acad Dermatol. 1998; S 87–94.

26. Ling MR, Swinger LJ, Jarratt MT et al. Once-weekly fluconazole (450 mg) for 4, 6, or 9 months of treatment for distal subungual onychomycosis of the toenail. J Am Acad Dermatol. 1998; S 95–102.

27. Fräki JE, Heikkilä HT et al. An open-label, noncomparative, multicenter evaluation of fluconazole with or without urea nail pedicure for treatment of onychomycosis. Curr Therap Res. 1997; 58: 481–491.

28. Ryder NS. Terbinafine: mode of action and properties of the squalene epoxidase inhibition. Br J Dermatol 1992; 126:2–7

29. Balfour JA, Faulds D. Terbinafine: a review of its pharmacodynamic and pharmacokinetic properties, and therapeutic potential in superficial mycoses. Drugs 1992; 43:259–284

30. Finlay AJ. Pharmacokinetics of terbinafine in the nail. Br J Dermatol 1992; 126:28–32

31. Faergemann J, Zehender H, Millerioux L. Levels of terbinafine in plasma, stratum corneum, dermisepidermis (without stratum corneum), sebum, hair and nails during and after 250 mg terbinafine orally once daily for 7 and 14 days. Clin Exp Dermatol 1994; 19:121–126

32. O'Sullivan DP, Needham CA, Bangs CA, Atkin K, Kendall FD. Postmarketing surveillance of oral terbinafine in the UK: report of a large cohort study. Br J Clin Pharmacol 1996; 42:559–565

33. Stricker BH, van Riemsdijk MM, Sturkenboom MC, Ottervanger JP. Taste loss to terbinafine: a case-control study of potential risk factors. Br J Clin Pharmacol 1996; 42:313–318

34. Vantaux P, Grasset D, Nougue J, Lagier E, Seigneuric C. Hépatite aiguë en rapport avec la prise de terbinafine. Gastroenterol Clin Biol 1996; 20:402–403

35. Rzany B, Mockenhaupt M, Gehring W, Schpf E. Stevens-Johnson syndrome after terbinafine therapy. J Am Acad Dermatol 1994; 30: 509

36. Carstens J, Wendelboe P, Sogaard H, Thestrup-Pedersen K. Toxic epidermal necrolysis and erythema multiforme following therapy with terbinafine. Acta Dermatol Venereol 1994; 74:391–392

37. Deutsches Ärzteblatt. 1997; 94: B 1695.

38. van der Schroeff JG, Cirkel PKS, Crijns MB et al. A randomized treatment duration-finding study of terbinafine in onychomycosis. Br J Dermatol 1992; 126:36–39

39. Svejgaard EL, Brandrup F, Kragballe K, Larsen PØ, Veien NK, Holst M, Andersen BL, Bro-Jörgensen AV, Dahl JC, Frentz G, Graudal C, Kamp P, Kroman N, Larsen FS, Mikkelsen F, Munkvad JM, Olafsson JH, Rothenborg H, Staberg D, Sondergaard J, Thulin H. Oral terbinafine in toenail dermatophytosis. A double-blind, placebo-controlled multicenter study with 12 months' follow-up. Acta Dermatol Venereol 1997; 77:66–69

40. Haneke E, Tausch I, Bräutigam M, Weidinger G, Welzel D, LAGOS III Study Group. Short-duration treatment of fingernail dermatophytosis: a randomized, double-blind study with terbinafine and griseofulvin. J Am Acad Dermatol 1995; 32:72–77

41. Arenas R, Dominguez-Cherit J, Fernandez LMA. Open randomized comparison of itraconazole versus terbinafine in onychomycosis. Int J Dermatol. 1995; 34: 138–143.

42. De Backer M, De Vroey C, Lesaffre E et al. Twelve weeks of continuous oral therapy for toenail onychomycosis caused by dermatophytes: a double-blind comparative trial of terbinafine 250 mg/day versus itraconazole 200 mg/day. J Am Acad Dermatol. 1998; 38: S 57–S 63.

43. Bräutigam M, Nolting S, Schopf RE, Weidinger G, Lagos VII Group. Randomized double blind comparison of terbinafine and itraconazole for treatment of toenail tinea infection. Br Med J 1995; 322: 919–922.

44. Tosti A, Piraccini BM, Stinchi C, Venturo N, Bardazzi F, Colombo MD. Treatment of dermatophyte nail infections: an open randomized study comparing intermittent terbinafine therapy with continuous terbinafine treatment and intermittent itraconazole therapy. J Am Acad 1996; 34:595–600

45. Billstein S, Evans EGU, Sigurgeirsson B. An analysis of the efficacy, safety, and tolerability of terbinafine versus pulsed itraconazole in the treatment of toenail onychomycosis. JEADV 1998; II (Supplement 2): 231–232

46. Feuilhade M, Baran R, Goettmann S, Pietrini P, Viguié C, Badillet G, Larnier C. Onychomycoses dermatophytiques avec atteinte de la matrice: Intérêt de l'association d'un vernis contenant 5% amorolfine à un traitement oral par terbinafine. Ann Dermatol Vénéréol 1996; 123: Suppl I:S143

47. Goodfield MJD, Bosanquet N, Evans EGV et al. Cost effective clinical management of onychomycosis. Br J Med Econ 1994; 7:15–23

7.3.1 Treatment in the elderly

In this type of patient, treatment must be individualized. It will depend on the patient's needs, physical condition, the site of the lesions (fingers or toes), any associated pathology (which might be multiple), the type of onychomycosis (onychogryphosis, for example) and the possibility of underlying vascular impairment. In elderly patients with trophic disorders of the legs, repeated isolation of *Candida ciferrii* from toenails was recently reported [1]. *Onychocola canadensis*, often involving all the toenails with a yellowish, slightly hyperkeratotic and markedly friable dystrophy, is probably also underestimated as an agent of onychomycosis in elderly individuals with arteriovenous problems associated with leg ulcers, because of the slow growth of the fungi in culture and the necessity for a subculture for identification [2]. Finally, the clinicopathological spectrum of foot disease may be related to wearing improperly fitting shoes.

A patient in good health can be treated in the same manner as a young adult. Nevertheless the management of finger and toenail diseases requires different considerations. The latter may require less medication but more chiropody. This may involve the abrasion of hyperkeratotic nails by means of a specially designed electric file with a pear-shaped, carbide bit.

It might be advisable to refrain from additional systemic treatment in patients who may already be taking several medications. However, if the patient is both insistent and distressed by the disease, one could consider a weekly dose of fluconazole (300 mg). With this exception, these patients should receive only local treatment such as chemical nail avulsion, which carries no risk to the ischaemic toe or antifungal nail lacquers [3]. Both offer an improvement in terms of patient compliance and results may also be improved as both approaches involve the use of assistance of a third person to apply properly the treatment.

Table 7.5
Adverse events of currently used systemic antifungals

	Itraconazole	Fluconazole	Terbinafine
Overall incidence	10–15 %	10–15 %	10 –15 %
Gastrointestinal	Nausea, vomiting, abdominal pain, diarrhoea, asymptomatic increase of liver enzymes	Nausea, vomiting, abdominal pain, diarrhoea, asymptomatic increase of liver enzymes	Nausea, vomiting, dyspepsia, diarrhoea, cramps, sickness, taste alterations
Skin	Rash, oedema, urticaria, generalized pustulosis	Rash, Stevens-Johnson syndrome, toxic epidermal necrolysis, fixed drug eruption	Rash, urticaria, serum-sickness-like reaction, eczema, erythroderma, Stevens-Johnson syndrome, toxic epidermal necrolysis
CNS	Headache, dizziness	Headache, seizure	Headache, dizziness, sleeplessness, green vision
Other	Hypokalaemia, thrombocytopenia plus leukopenia, drug interactions	Agranulocytosis, thrombocytopenia, adrenal insufficiency, congenital anomalies	Pancytopenia

7.3.2 Treatment in childhood [4-5]

Children with onychomycosis should be carefully examined for concomitant tinea capitis and tinea pedis. Their parents and siblings should also be checked for onychomycosis and tinea pedis.

Topical formulations, using transungual anti-fungal delivery system and bifonazole in a 40% urea cream are suitable first treatment options. If systemic treatment is necessary, as in adults, it will require 6 weeks of continuous terbinafine therapy for the fingers and 3 months for the toes. The dose suggested would be 250 mg/day when the weight exceeds 40 kg; 125 mg/day at a weight of 20 to 40 kg and 62.5 mg/daily for children weighing less than 20 kg. With itraconazole pulsed therapy (2 weeks over 2 months for fingernails and 3 weeks over 3 months for toenails, the doses suggested would be 200 mg/twice daily when the weight exceeds 50 kg ; 200 mg/day at a weight of 40 to 50 kg ; 100 mg/day at a weight of 20 to 40 kg and 5 mg/kg daily for children weighing less than 20 kg; an oral solution is available (3 mg/kg/day) [6].

Intermittent therapy with fluconazole requires a weekly 3 to 6 mg/kg single dose for 12-16 weeks for fingernails, 18-26 weeks for the toe-nails (a suspension is available).

As none of these antifungals is approved for use in dermatophyte onychomycoses in children in all countries, clinical judgement is needed to assess the potential benefits and risks to the patient. In onychomycosis, some advise carrying out blood tests every 8 weeks including electrolyte levels (itraconazole, fluco-nazole); liver function tests (all drugs) and complete blood count with a differential (all drugs) [5].

7.3.3 Treatment in pregnant women

There is only limited experience in the use of itraconazole in pregnancy, but it can penetrate the blood–placenta barrier. Due to its lipophilicity, it is excreted in breast-milk and breast-feeding women are therefore advised not to take this drug.

Fluconazole has been associated with con-genital anomalies and should therefore not be given to pregnant women.

There is no evidence of an interaction between oral terbinafine and oral contraceptives, and oral terbinafine does not appear to affect the outcome of pregnancy [7]. Clinical experience with terbinafine during pregnancy is, however, minimal.

According to FDA pregnancy categories, these new systemic antifungal agents have been classified as follows: itraconazole and fluco-nazole belong to category C and terbinafine to category B. However, it is generally prudent to avoid using any of these drugs in pregnant women.

7.3.4 Treatment in immunocompromised patients

Onychomycosis is frequently seen in HIV-infected patients, and several studies have reported prevalence rates of up to 12% [8]. In AIDS patients onychomycosis can be observed without evidence of dermatophytosis else-where on the skin [9]. Onychomycosis com-monly appears when the CD4 cell count is less than 450 cells/mm^3 [10]. Tinea unguium corre-lates with disease progression. Generalized chronic dermatophytosis has been reported in subjects with CD4 lymphocyte counts of less than 200/mm^3 [11].

The same fungal infections commonly seen in the HIV-negative population are also seen among HIV-positive individuals, and the same effective antifungal agents are generally useful although relapse rates are higher [12]. Besides physical discomfort, fungal nail infection can cause profound emotional distress for patients with HIV infection and serve as a daily reminder of a disease that might otherwise still be asymptomatic.

Onychomycosis due to dermatophytes is frequent and *T. rubrum* is the most commonly isolated organism which may even involve periungual tissues. PSO represents 90% of the cases of onychomycosis in AIDS. In immunosuppressed patients, onycho-mycoses due to non-dermatophytes account for only a small proportion of the cases. *Fusarium* spp. may be dangerous in neutro-penic patients because the toenail can be a possible portal of entry for systemic infection which can be rapidly fatal despite institution of amphotericin B therapy [13] which has the highest in vitro activity and should be currently considered as the treatment of choice[14].

Immunocompromised patients present special therapeutic problems ranging from failure to eradicate the organism completely, toxicity, and replacement of the most common *Candida* species with others more resistant to treatment such as *Candida glabrata* [15]. The develop-ment of yeast resistance in immunocompromi-sed patients is beginning to prove a significant difficulty, especially in AIDS cases [16]. In addi-tion, these patients tend to have more severe disease with frequent recurrences [17].

References

1. de Gentile L, Bouchara JP, Le Clec'h C et al. Prevalence of *Candida ciferrii* in elderly patients with trophic disor-ders of the legs. Mycopathologia 1995; 131: 99–102.

2. Contet-Audonneau N, Schmutz JL, Basile AM et al. A new agent of ony-chomycosis in elderly: *Onychocola canadensis.* Eur J Dermatol.1997; 7: 115–117.

3. Seebacher C, Ulbricht H, Würz K. Topical therapy of onychomycoses in geriatric patients. TW Dermatol. 1993; 23: 434–438.

4. Gupta AK, Sibbald RG, Lynde CW et al. Onychomycosis in children. Prevalence and treatment strategies. J Am Acad Dermatol. 1997; 36: 395–402.

5. Suarez S. New antifungal therapy for children. In: James WD, Cockerell J, Dzubow LM et al. (eds). Advances in Dermatology 1997; 12: 195–209.

6. Gupta AK, Chang P, del Rosso DV et al. Itraconazole for the treatment of onychomycosis in children. Poster 202 – AAD 1998 – Orlando.

7. Williams TG, Hall M. Lack of inter-action of oral terbinafine with oral contraceptives and healthy babies in a postmarketing surveillance study. Fifth annual international summit on cutaneous antifungal therapy. Abstract 67. Singapore, 1998.

8. Sindrup JH, Weismann K, Petersen CS et al. Skin and oral mucosal changes in patients infected with human immunodeficiency virus. Acta Derm Venereol. 1988; 68: 440–443.

9. Ravnborg L, Baastrup N, Svejgaard E. Onychomycosis in HIV-infected patients. Acta Derm Venereol 1998; 78: 151–152.

10. Gregory N. Special populations: onychomycosis in the HIV-positive patient. J Am Acad Dermatol 1996; 35: S13–S16.

11. Goldman GD, Bolognia JL. HIV-related skin disease: managing fungal infections. J Respir. Dis. 1997; 18: 14–20.

12. Herranz P, Garcia J, De Lucas R et al. Toenail onychomycosis in patients with acquired immune deficiency syndrome: treatment with terbinafine. Br J Dermatol 1997; 139: 577–580.

13. Arrese JE, Piérard-Franchimont C, Piérard GE. Fatal hyalohyphomycosis following Fusarium onychomycosis in an immunocompromised patient. Am J Dermatopathol. 1996; 18: 196–198.

14. Martino P, Gastaldi R, Raccah R, et al. Clinical patterns of Fusarium infections in immunocompromised patients. J Infect. 1994; 28: suppl 1: 7–15.

15. Evans EGV. Causative pathogens in onychomycosis and the possibility of treatment resistance: A review. J Am Acad Dermatol. 1998; 38: S 32–36.

16. Roberts DT. Cutaneous candidosis. Dermatol Therapy. 1997; 3: 26–36.

17. Lemak NA, Duvic M. Superficial fungal infections in HIV and AIDS. Dermatol Therapy. 1997; 3: 84–90.

7.4 Rationale for a stepwise approach to therapy

Besides the five main considerations for choosing a drug (efficacy, safety, cost, compliance, and availability [1]), choice of treatment (Fig 7.32) depends on many factors including patient's age and preference, infecting fungus, number of nails affected, degree of nail involvement, whether toenails or fingernails are infected, and whether other drugs are taken [2]. In order to improve on efficacy, some investigators still suggest that one management approach would be to check mycological status six months after the start of systemic therapy and then to repeat treatment for those with positive results with the same antifungal (terbinafine [3-4] or itraconzole [5]), or with fluconazole after a course of terbinafine [6]. However, by following such strategies we probably move away from one of the considerations of great importance nowadays, i.e. cost effectiveness [7].

Sequential pulse therapy for fingernail onychomycosis, with itraconazole (200 mg twice daily for one week), was followed 3 weeks later by a pulse of terbinafine (25 mg twice daily for one week). Patients were evaluated 4 months from the start of treatment, and if necessary it was supplemented with another pulse of itraconazole only. All patients were cured [7a].

It is important to recognize that fungal invasion of certain sites e.g. the lunula, the lateral edge of the nail and the subungual area (which may lead to extensive onycholysis) may affect recovery. Therefore, a rationale for a staged-therapy approach in treating onychomycosis is suggested [7b] (Fig 7.33).

Early infections with involvement of the distal $\frac{2}{3}$ of the nail plate of up to two to four digits may be treated with topical monotherapy using the nail lacquers that act as transungual drug delivery systems. The shorter the length of nail plate invasion, the better the treatment response. Such treatment of distal subungual onychomycosis at the beginning of the fungal invasive process solves the problem of

Fig 7.32
Onychomycosis
Therapeutic options

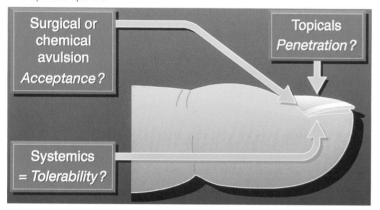

Fig 7.33
Rational treatment of onychomycosis
Which route to follow in different stages?

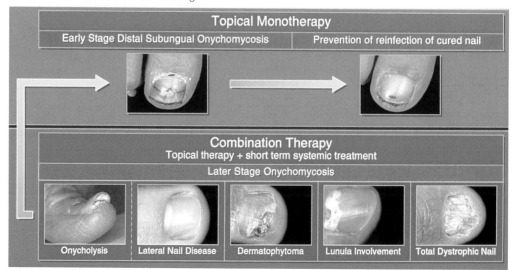

retaining the active agent in contact with the substrate for long enough to produce the desired antifungal action. Should there be no significant clinical success after a period of six months, a short course with systemic antifungal agents should be added.

Topical monotherapy is ineffective in more extensive infections including those with the local factors already mentioned, i.e. where the nail plate is no longer in contact with the subungual tissue (as this interrupts the transport of the drug from the nail into the nail bed). Equally, this drawback is also encountered with the new systemic antifungal drugs which usually penetrate the nail via the nail bed, thereby interrupting the transport process of the drug from the nail bed into the ventral nail plate (Fig 7.34). Even though these drugs still enter the nail keratin through the matrix, the clinical and mycological response may be diminished. One potential solution to the management of these more extensive infections involves using antifungal nail lacquer and oral therapy with one of the newer drugs e.g. terbinafine [8], itraconazole [9] or fluconazole from the start. The use of combined topical and systemic therapy may be expensive, but since the cure rate is higher, the overall cost of therapy is reduced. In countries where this is not an issue, it is a logical clinical choice in some infections.

This combination is potentially beneficial since topical treatment may eradicate fungal foci in the nail plate and systemic antifungals treat the nail bed and tinea pedis which usually precedes onychomycosis. Chemical or partial surgical nail avulsion may also be used to supplement the treatment to eliminate the factors

Fig 7.34
Extensive onycholysis

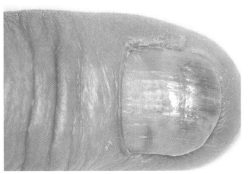

Fig 7.35
Action of antifungals on sterol biosynthesis

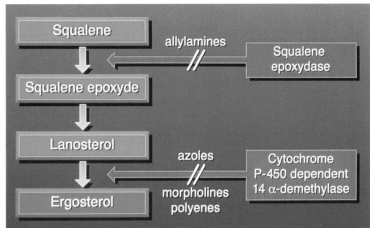

encouraging chronicity such as the development of irregularities of the nail bed. Such a combination also minimizes the risk of adverse effects from systemic drugs which might have to be given for a long period.

Antifungal combinations may increase the magnitude and rate of microbial killing in vivo, shorten the total duration of therapy, prevent the emergence of drug resistance, expand the spectrum of activity, and decrease drug-related toxicity by using lower doses of systemic antifungals [10, 11, 12].

Biochemical studies have identified a number of potential targets for antifungal chemotherapy, including cell wall synthesis, membrane sterol biosynthesis (Fig 7.35), nucleic acid synthesis, metabolic inhibition and macromolecular biosynthesis [11]. The inhibition of cell wall synthesis would be, in theory, highly specific since only fungal cells build their cell wall with chitin and glucan. Since the modern systemic azoles and allylamines as well as the topical amorolfine act very specifically on the ergosterol biosynthesis in the cell membrane, as a rational partner for combination therapy one may prefer to combine the new systemic drugs with ciclopirox which acts by a completely different mechanism (Fig 7.36). As yet there is no suitable preparation of the new cell wall antagonists such as the echinocandins, currently in development.

Fig 7.36
Potential targets of antifungal agents (after A. Polak)

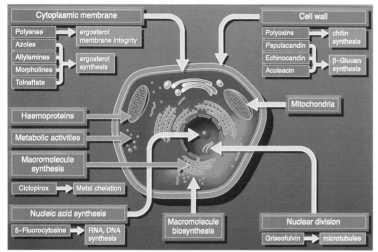

Other therapeutic problems

1) Isolated onycholysis associated with
   Candida spp.

2) Chronic paronychia

3) Non-dermatophyte moulds

Onycholysis associated with *Candida* spp.
[13]
Isolated onycholysis associated with *Candida*
spp. often coexists with bacterial infection
(Pseudomonas or *Proteus)* [14]. The nail has to
be trimmed back as far as possible (local anaesthesia may be required for anxious patients),
the nail bed should be debrided with a piece of
gauze wrapped around a stick. A topical agent
such as ciclopirox or clotrimazole must be
applied daily. However, unless there is morpho-
logical or histological evidence of nail plate
invasion, the fungi are generally found colon-
izing the ventral nail plate and onycholysis must
be managed separately.

Chronic paronychia
The proper treatment of chronic paronychia
cannot be generalized since it requires the
identification of different aetiological factors
responsible for the condition [13, 15].
Patients need precise counselling about the

environmental hazards that may exacerbate
their condition, such as "wet occupation"
(e.g. kitchen work) and microtrauma.

Patients with irritative chronic paronychia or
with contact allergy, food hypersensitivity, or
Candida hypersensitivity greatly improve with
the daily application of potent topical steroids.
In severe cases intralesional injections or
systemic steroids can be used.

If *Candida* is present a topical imidazole
derivative or ciclopirox cream can supplement
the steroid treatment. Solutions are a preferable
treatment, as they penetrate to the site of
infection better. Systemic antifungals are not
more useful, except in true *Candida* paronychia
infection.

Chronic paronychia can be considered cured
only when the cuticle has completely regrown.

In recalcitrant cases of chronic paronychia due
to foreign bodies (in hairdressers for example)
a crescent of thickened nail fold may be
excised under regional block anaesthesia.
Complete healing by secondary intention and
restoration of the proximal nail fold with
adherent cuticle takes place in less than one
month.

Non-dermatophyte moulds
SWO caused by non-dermatophyte moulds
may respond to abrasion of the nail surface
followed by topical therapy with imidazole
agents, amorolfine or ciclopirox.

In the other clinical patterns, non-dermatophyte
moulds are most likely to be contaminating
organisms in onychomycosis due to dermatophytes, secondary to the dermatophyte.
Removal of the other fungi does not influence
the outcome of treatment [16].

DLSO associated with only non-dermatophyte
moulds such as *Aspergillus* spp., *Fusarium*
spp., *Sytalidium* spp., *Scopulariopsis brevicaulis* and *Alternaria* spp. may respond
to intermittent itraconazole therapy [17] or to
systemic terbinafine [18]. However best results
may be obtained when systemic antifungals
may be associated with topical treatment
preceded by surgical or chemical nail avulsion
[19].

Table 7.6

Causes of failure of onychomycosis treatment (After poster 187 AAD 1998, modified) [20].

1. Poor compliance

2. Misdiagnosis
   - laboratory tests neglected
   - dual pathology
   - bacterial association [14]

3. Dietary mistakes (itraconazole and ketoconazole intake)
   - reduced gastric acidity/achlorhydria (for example in AIDS or neutropenia patients) should be compensated by intake with acidic fruit juice
   - empty stomach, since resorption of these drugs (as well as griseofulvin) are influenced by presence of fat-containing meal.

4. Clinical variants
   - extensive onycholysis
   - lateral nail fungal infection
   - dermatophytoma
   - paronychia

5. Mycological variants
   - presence of arthroconidia with thicker cell walls [20]
   - dematiaceous fungi

– *Trichophyton rubrum nigricans* [20]
– development of yeast resistance in immunocompromised patients as well as replacement of the most common *Candida* spp with others more resistant to treatment [22].

6. Bioavailability of drug interactions (see text)

7. Local factors
   - reduced linear nail growth
   - wearing improperly fitted shoes

8. Systemic factors
   - peripheral circulation impairment
   - endocrine diseases (diabetes, Cushing)
   - ageing with multiple associated factors

9. Host response
   - Endogenous immunologic factors
     AIDS, CMCC
     Chronic dermatophytosis
   - Exogenous immunologic factors
     Immunosuppressive therapy (transplant patients)
     Chemotherapy

References

1. Gupta AK, Scher RK, de Doncker P. Current management of onychomycosis. Dermatol Clinics. 1997; 15: 121–135.

2. Denning DW, Evans EG, Kibbler CC et al. Fungal nail disease: a guide to good practice. BMJ, 1995; 311: 1271–1281.

3. Tausch I, Bräutigam M, Weiding G. Evaluation of 6 weeks treatment of terbinafine in tinea unguium in a double-blind trial comparing 6 and 12 weeks therapy. Br J Dermatol 1997; 136: 737–742.

4. Watson A, Marley J, Ellis D et al. Terbinafine in onychomycosis of the toenail: a novel treatment protocol. J Am Acad Dermatol. 1995; 33: 775–779.

5. Haneke E, Ring J, Abeck D. Efficacy of itraconazole pulse treatment in onychomycosis. H-G-Z- Hautkr. 1997; 72: 737–740.

6. De Cuyper C. Therapeutic approach of recalcitrant toenail onychomycosis. Fifth Internatiional Summit on Cutaneous Antifungal Therapy. Abstract 26. Singapore 1998.

7. Einarson TR, Oh PI, Shear NH. Multinational pharmacoeconomic analysis of topical and oral therapies for onychomycosis. J. Dermatol Treat 1997; 8 (Iss. 4): 229–235.

7a. Gupta AK, Konnikov N, Lynde CW. Sequential pulse therapy with itraconazole and terbinafine to treat onychomycosis of the fingernails. J Dermatological Treat 2000; 11: 151–154.

7b. Baran R. Differential diagnosis of onychomycosis and rationale for a step therapy in treating nail fungal infection. In: Shuster S (ed). Hydroxy-pyridones as antifungal agents with special emphasis on onychomycosis. Chap 17: 103–109. Berlin, Springer, 1999.

8. Baran R, Feuilhade M, Datry A et al. A randomized trial of amorolfine 5% solution nail lacquer combined with oral terbinafine compared with terbinafine alone in the treatment of dermatophytic toenail onychomycoses affecting the matrix region. Br J Dermatol 2000; 142: 1177–1183.

9. Nolting S. Open studies of ciclopirox nail lacquer in onychomycosis – A review. In: Schuster S (ed). Hydroxy-pyridones as antifungal agents with special emphasis on onychomycosis. Chap 13: 75–80. Berlin, Springer, 1999.

10. Ghannoum MA. Future of antimycotic therapy. Dermatol Therapy. 1997; 3:104–111.

11. Polak-Wyss A. Mechanism of action of antifungals and combination therapy. J Eur Acad Dermatol Venereol. 1995; 4, suppl. 1: 511–516)

12. Polak A. Combination therapy for systemic mycosis. Infection 1996; 17: 203–209.

13. Daniel CR, Daniel MP, Daniel CM et al. Chronic paronychia and onycholysis: a thirteen-year experience. Cutis 1996; 58: 397–401.

14. Elewski BE. Bacterial infection in a patient with onychomycosis. J Am Acad Dermatol. 1997; 37: 493–494.

15. Tosti A, Piraccini BM. Paronychia. In Amin S, Maibach H. (eds). Contact urticaria syndrome. CRC Press S. Boca Raton USA, 1997. Chap 26, p 276–278.

16. Ellis DH, Marley JE, Watson AB. Significance of non-dermatophyte moulds and yeasts in onychomycosis. Dermatology 1997;194 (suppl 1): 40–42.

17. de Doncker P, Scher RK, Baran R et al. Itraconazole therapy is effective for pedal onychomycosis caused by some non dermatophyte molds and in mixed infection by dermatophytes and molds. A multicenter study with 36 patients. J Am Acad Dermatol. 1997;36:173–177.

18. Nolting S, Brautigam M, Weidinger G. Terbinafine in onychomycosis with involvement by non-dermatophytic fungi. Br J Derm. 1994, 130: suppl 43: 16–21.

19. Tosti A, Piraccini BM. Treatment of onychomycosis: a European experience. Dermatol Therapy. 1997; 3: 66–72.

20. de Doncker P, Degreef H, André J, Pierard G. Why are some with onychomycosis still not responding to the newer antifungal agents? Poster 187. AAD, 1998, Orlando.

21. Perrin Ch, Baran R. Longitudinal melanonychia caused by Trichophyton rubrum. J Am Acad Dermatol. 1994; 31: 311–316.

22. Roberts DT. Cutaneous candidosis. Dermatol Therapy. 1997; 3: 26–36.

There is an excellent therapeutic response to terbinafine (82% clinical cure or with minimal residual lesions and 82% mycological cure after 2 years) [1–3]. However, in some patients with onychomycosis, treated with the new systemic antifungals, the long term results are somewhat disappointing, but definitely better with terbinafine [3a], especially in patients followed for 5 years after initiation of original treatment with terbinafine or itraconazole [3b].

A study reports on the 3 year follow-up of a group of 47 'cured' patients with toenail onychomycosis. They were treated with a 4 month course of either terbinafine or itraconazole. Relapses were more common in patients treated with pulsed itraconazole (36.3 %) than in patients treated with continuous (16.6%) or intermittent (15.3%) terbinafine [4]. This was confirmed in a double blind comparative trial of terbinafine 250 mg/day versus itraconazole 200 mg/day for 12 weeks [5].

In another study of 88 patients, 36 weeks after cessation of 12 weeks' itraconazole (continuous or pulse) therapy, total clinical cure was achieved in 35% of these patients with 93% negative culture. At a follow-up at week 104 the total clinical cure was 39%, with negative culture in 57%. Younger patients showed significantly better clinical cure rates at week 36 than older patients. This could be due to the faster nail growth in young people [6]. A group of patients treated with 250 mg terbinafine daily for 3 to 6 months was followed for approximately 2½ years. Although some patients changed status from cured to not cured and vice versa, nearly half of the patients

had a clinical cure after 1 year and a clinical and mycological cure after 2½ years [7].

Moreover, Epstein investigated how often oral treatment of toenail onychomycosis does produce a disease-free nail and concludes that this goal is achieved with standard courses of terbinafine in approximately 35%–50% of patients. For itraconazole, the relevant disease-free nail rate was about 25%–40%. He also stated that disease reappearance is an important issue and that corresponding data are unfortunately still missing [8].

This statement leads spontaneously to the question as to whether efficacious prophylactic treatment is necessary and possible. In this context the application of the new topical transungual drug delivery systems should be investigated since systemic treatment for prophylactic use cannot be justified due to possible side effects, drug interactions and high costs.

8.1 Reasons for prevention

These studies suggest that the long term outlook for some patients receiving treatment for fungal nail disease is unsatisfactory because of treatment failure, relapse or reinfection.

Failure of treatment of onychomycosis may be due to reinfection or to incomplete eradication of the original fungus with treatment (recurrence) (See Table 7.6). Although in most cases it is virtually impossible to distinguish reinfections from true relapses. Failures that occur within 1 year after interruption of treatment are more likely to be recurrences, whereas failures that occur later are probably reinfections. The latter probably accounts for about ⅔ of relapses [2]. This raises the question as to why patients with onychomycosis are so easily reinfected. Susceptibility to onychomycosis depends on several factors, including genetic predisposition, reduced nail growth rate and underlying disease.

8.1.1 Genetic predisposition

Trichophyton rubrum onychomycosis frequently occurs in several members of the same family in different generations (Fig 8. 1). *Trichophyton rubrum* infection, however, is rare in persons marrying into infected families, suggesting a genetic predisposition rather than an intrafamilial transmission of the infection. It is

Fig 8.1
Genetic predisposition to *T. rubrum*

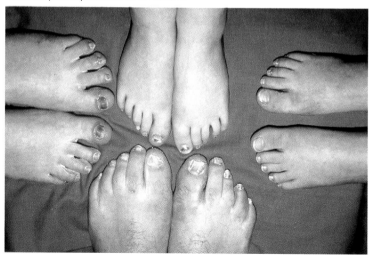

Courtesy DT Roberts (Glasgow)

associated with atopy, for instance [9]. Pedigree studies suggest an autosomal dominant inheritance [10]. According to Zaias, predisposed individuals acquire *Trichophyton rubrum* infection in early childhood from their infected parents. The infection remains localized to the plantar region for many years without being noticed by the patient. Nail invasion, which usually begins in adult life, is possibly favoured by local factors such as reduced nail growth rate and trauma. Genetic predisposition to *T. rubrum* invasion may possibly be linked to biochemical abnormalities in the keratins. A genetic susceptibility to infection by *T. concentricum* (tinea imbricata) has also been suggested.

Gender has a role in determining the risk that an individual will develop onychomycosis [11, 12]. In one survey, the risk of males having onychomycosis was 84.3% greater than for females of the same age [11].

8.1.2 Reduced nail growth rate

It has been suggested that onychomycosis affects the toenails of elderly individuals because of slow growth rate [13], a hypothesis which is still debatable (see p. 41).

8.1.3 Underlying disease
Nail diseases

Onycholysis and nail bed hyperkeratosis may favour nail invasion by fungi. This explains why onychomycosis is quite common in patients with traumatic nail dystrophies or nail bed psoriasis [14].

Dermatological diseases

Dermatophyte infection is often observed in patients with palmoplantar keratoderma or ichthyosis [15, 16].

Systemic disease

Peripheral vascular disorders and diabetes mellitus have frequently been reported to predispose to onychomycosis [17]. However, recent epidemiological data are against the association between onychomycosis and diabetes [18], although the majority of patients in this study had type I diabetes mellitus, affecting a younger age group who are less prone to onychomycosis. Other endocrine diseases (Cushing's syndrome [19], metabolic disorders, peripheral neuropathies and lymphoma [20]) have also been considered as predisposing factors.

Immunosuppression clearly predisposes to onychomycosis, and nail invasion by yeasts is almost exclusively seen in patients with impaired immune function.

Patients with HIV infection are more commonly affected by onychomycosis than healthy individuals [21]. In these patients onychomycosis is frequently caused by fungi that do not usually invade nails of immunocompetent individuals, such as *Candida* spp. and *Fusarium* spp. In some cases nail infection may represent the portal of entry for a disseminated infection. Proximal subungual onychomycosis due to *T. rubrum* is often observed in HIV-positive patients, where it is considered to be a negative prognostic feature. For this reason, patients with *T. rubrum* proximal subungual onychomycosis should be examined for the presence of underlying immunosuppression.

8.2 Prevention

Since relapses of onychomycosis are frequent, consideration should be given to prevention of reccurrences in patients who have been cured. High rates of infections have been associated with working conditions where:
– workers are required to wear heavy duty shoes which create a confined, damp and warm atmosphere that facilitates the development of fungal and bacterial infections.
– industries do not provide sufficient information to workers about the importance of foot hygiene.
– jobs necessitate the use of communal showers, which can lead to recurrent fungal contamination.

Collective preventive measures

These are generally ineffective because they are difficult to apply and/or not adhered to . **Ideally** the following situations are desirable [22]:
– tiled shower floors should be inclined to allow sufficient drainage and non-stagnation of wastewater *(Trichophyton rubrum* survives 25 days in stagnant water at 23–25°C).
– wooden shower-floor grids should be replaced by plastic ones to limit the adhesion of scales shed by infected feet.
– floors of communal showers must be washed and disinfected at least once daily with, for example, sodium hypochlorite, if possible after use by each group of workers.

Preventive Measures

Table 8.1
Individuals at risk

Armed forces, police	Mine workers
Athletes	Rubber-industry workers
Dustmen	Sewer workers
Employees of indoor swimming pools	Steel and furnace workers
Excavation workers	Wood-cutters

Individual preventive measures, have to be added to the collective preventive measures.

There is no evidence that disinfecting shoes and socks, though logical, affects the course or relapse rate of onychomycosis. It is, however, important to treat recurrent tinea pedis at the earliest opportunity. In individuals at risk for tinea pedis (Table 8.1) it is important to limit spread in shower rooms by providing disposable slippers and by careful foot hygiene including drying web spaces after showering. Tolnaftate [23], fenticonazole [24], ciclopiroxol-amine and bifonazole powder [25] have all been used prophylactically to prevent recurrent tinea pedis. A weekly application of terbinafine cream in the nail area [26], between the toes and on the soles of the feet would also be expected to be very effective in preventing reinfection in those individuals who appear to be particularly susceptible to onychomycosis.

Finally, long-term intermittent therapy might prevent the re-establishment of tinea pedis and limit the risk of nail reinfection. Periodic use of transungual antifungal drug delivery systems, which are retained in nail keratin after discontinuation of therapy, appears to be a logical and safe method for preventing recurrences but this needs confirmation in a large population. However it is doubtful if such approaches are practicable in the majority of patients and good foot hygiene at home or in the work place coupled with early treatment of recurrent tinea pedis may provide the best solution.

References

1. De Cuyper C. Long-term evaluation of terbinafine 250 and 500 mg daily in a 16-week oral treatment for toenail onychomycosis. Br J Dermatol. 1996; 135: 156.

2. De Baker M, De Vroey C, Lesaffre E et al. Twelve weeks of continuous oral therapy for toenail onychomycosis caused dermatophytes: a double-blind comparative trial of terbinafine 250 mg/day, versus itraconazole 200 mg/day. J Am Acad Dermatol. 1998; 38: S 57–63.

3. Bräutigam M. Terbinafine versus itraconazole: A controlled clinical comparison in onychomycosis of the toenails. J Am Acad Dermatol. 1998; 38: S 53–56.

3a. Evans EGV, Sigurgeirsson B (for the LION study group). Double blind, randomised study of continuous terbinafine compared with intermittent itraconazole in treatment of toenail onychomycosis. Br Med J 1999; 318: 1031–1035.

3b. Sigurgeirsson B. Long-term effectiveness of terbinafine vs itraconazole in onychomycosis: results of the LION Icelandic extension study (SS02–03). JEADV 2000; 14 (suppl 1): 82–83.

4. Tosti A, Piraccini BM, Stinchi C et al. Relapses of onychomycosis after successful treatment with systemic antifungals: a three year follow-up. Dermatology 1998; 197: 162–166.

5. De Backer M, De Vroey C, Lesaffre E et al. Twelve weeks of continuous oral therapy for toenail onychomycosis caused by dermatophytes: a double-blind comparative trial of terbinafine 250 mg/day versus itraconazole 200 mg/day. J Am Acad Dermatol. 1998; 38: S 57–63.

6. Heikkilä H, Stubb S. Long-term results of patients with onychomycosis treated with itraconazole. Acta Derm Venereol 1997; 77: 70–71.

7. Brandrup F Larsen PO. Long-term follow-up of toenail onychomycosis treated with terbinafine. Acta Derm Venereol. 1997; 77: 238.

8. Eppstein E. How often does oral treatment of toenail onychomycosis produce a disease-free nail? Arch Dermatol 1998; 134: 1551–1554.

9. Hanifin JM, Ray LF, Lobtiz WC. Immunological reactivity in dermatophytosis. Br J Dermatol 1974; 90: 1–8.

10. Zaias N, Tosti A, Rebell G et al. Autosomal dominant pattern of distal subungual onychomycosis caused by Trichophyton rubrum. J Am Acad Dermatol. 1996; 34: 302–304.

11. Gupta AK, Jain HC, Lynd CW et al. Prevalence and epidemiology of unsuspected onychomycosis in patients visiting dermatologists offices in Ontario, Canada. A multicenter survey of 2001 patients. Int J Derm 1998; 36: 783–787.

12. Elewski BE, Charif MA. Prevalence of onychomycosis in patients attending a dermatology clinic in northeastern Ohio for other conditions. Arch Dermatol 1997; 133: 1172–1173.

13. Orentreich N, Markofsky JV, Ogelman JH. The effect of aging on the rate of linear nail growth. J Invest Dermatol. 1979; 73: 126–130.

14. Gupta AK, Lynde CQ, Jain HC et al. A higher prevalence of onychomycosis in psoriatics compared with non-psoriatics: a multicentre study. Br J Dermatol. 1997; 136: 786.

15. Nielsen PG, Faergemann J. Dermatophytes and keratin in patients with hereditary palmoplantar keratoderma. Acta Derm Venereol. 1993; 73: 416–418.

16. Hay RJ. Chronic dermatophyte infections. Clinical and mycological features. Br J Dermatol. 1982; 106: 1–7.

17. Gupta AK, Konnikov N, MacDonald P et al. Prevalence of onychomycosis in diabetics: A North American Survey. Abstract .JEADV 1998.

18. Buxton PK, Milne LJR, Prescott RJ et al. The prevalence of dermatophyte infection in well-controlled diabetics and the response to Trichophyton antigen. Br J Dermatol. 1996; 134: 900–903.

19. Nelson LM, Mc Niece KJ. Recurrent Cushing's syndrome with Trichophyton rubrum infection. Arch Derm 1959; 85: 700–704.

20. Lewis GM, Hopper ME, Scott MJ. Generalised Trichophyton rubrum infection associated with systemic lymphoblastoma. Arch Derm 1953; 6: 247–262.

21. Daniel III CR, Norton LA, Scher RK. The spectrum of nail disease in patients with human immunodeficiency virus infection. J Am Acad Dermatol. 1992; 27: 93–97.

22. Baran R. Onychomycosis in: Epidemiology, Causes and Prevention of Skin diseases. Grob JJ, Stern RS, MacKie RM, Weinstock WA (eds) 1997 Blackwell, Oxford, Chp 15, p 276–278.

23. Smith EB, Dickson JE, Knox JM. Tolnaftate powder in prophylaxis of tinea pedis. South Med J. 1974; 67: 776–778.

24. Albanese G, Cintio R, Giorgetti P et al. Recurrent tinea pedis: a double blind study on the prophylactic use of fenticonazole powder. Mycoses 1992; 35: 157–159.

25. Galimberti RL, Belli L, Negroni R et al. Prophylaxis of tinea pedis interdigitalis with bifonazole. 1% powder. Dermatologica 1984; 169 suppl 1: 111–116.

26. Evans EG, Seaman RA, James IG. Short-duration therapy with terbinafine 1% cream in dermatophyte skin infections. Br J Dermatol. 1994; 130: 83–87.

Index

Index